The International Library of Bioethics

Volume 91

The *International Library of Bioethics* – formerly known as the International Library of Ethics, Law and the New Medicine comprises volumes with an international and interdisciplinary focus on foundational and applied issues in bioethics. With this renewal of a successful series we aim to meet the challenge of our time: how to direct biotechnology to human and other living things' ends, how to deal with changed values in the areas of religion, society, and culture, and how to formulate a new way of thinking, a new bioethics.

The *International Library of Bioethics* focuses on the role of bioethics against the background of increasing globalization and interdependency of the world's cultures and governments, with mutual influencing occurring throughout the world in all fields. The series will continue to focus on perennial issues of aging, mental health, preventive medicine, medical research issues, end of life, biolaw, and other areas of bioethics, whilst expanding into other current and future topics.

We welcome book proposals representing the broad interest of this series' interdisciplinary and international focus. We especially encourage proposals addressing aspects of changes in biological and medical research and clinical health care, health policy, medical and biotechnology, and other applied ethical areas involving living things, with an emphasis on those interventions and alterations that force us to re-examine foundational issues.

More information about this series at https://link.springer.com/bookseries/16538

Nanette Elster · Kayhan Parsi
Editors

Transitioning to Adulthood with Autism: Ethical, Legal and Social Issues

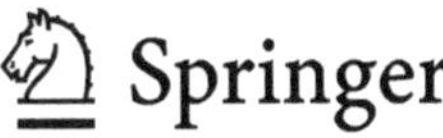

Editors
Nanette Elster
Neiswanger Institute for Bioethics
Loyola University Chicago Stritch School of Medicine
Maywood, IL, USA

Kayhan Parsi
Neiswanger Institute for Bioethics
Loyola University Chicago Stritch School of Medicine
Maywood, IL, USA

ISSN 2662-9186 ISSN 2662-9194 (electronic)
The International Library of Bioethics
ISBN 978-3-030-91486-8 ISBN 978-3-030-91487-5 (eBook)
https://doi.org/10.1007/978-3-030-91487-5

This Springer imprint is published by the registered company Springer Nature Switzerland AG
The registered company address is: Gewerbestrasse 11, 6330 Cham, Switzerland

We want to dedicate this book to Allanah and Gabriel, who inspire us to understand them and their interior worlds every day and who have broadened our understanding of the value neurodiversity brings. We also want to dedicate this to Dominic, who has spent his neurotypical life immersed in the world of neurodiversity.

Contents

Contributors

Haley J. Bishop Center for Injury Research and Prevention at CHOP, Philadelphia, PA, USA

Allison E. Curry Center for Injury Research and Prevention at CHOP, Philadelphia, PA, USA

Nathan Derhammer Loyola University Medical Center, Maywood, IL, USA

Cavan Doyle AMITA Health, Chicago, IL, USA

Lawrence A. Dubin University of Detroit Mercy, Detroit, MI, USA

Allanah Elster Columbia University, New York, NY, USA

Nanette Elster Neiswanger Institute for Bioethics, Loyola University Chicago Stritch School of Medicine, Maywood, IL, USA

Laurie Gutmann Kahn Moravian College, Bethlehem, PA, USA

Marisa Kofke Moravian College, Bethlehem, PA, USA

Katrine Krause-Jensen School of Culture and Society, Aarhus University, Aarhus, Denmark

Ellen Parker Loyola University Medical Center, Maywood, IL, USA

Kayhan Parsi Neiswanger Institute for Bioethics, Loyola University Chicago Stritch School of Medicine, Maywood, IL, USA

Lillian Peterson Giant Steps, Lisle, IL, USA

Kenneth A. Richman Center for Health Humanities, MCPHS University, Boston, MA, USA

Raffaele Rodogno School of Culture and Society, Aarhus University, Aarhus, Denmark

Rita Rossi-Foulkes Department of Medicine (Medicine-Pediatrics), University of Chicago, Chicago, IL, USA

Eugene Schnitzler Loyola University Medical Center, Maywood, IL, USA

Angelina Strum Giant Steps, Lisle, IL, USA

Moshe Weitzberg Aspiritech NFP, Highwood, IL, USA

Elizabeth M. Yang WStrong, LLC, Reston, VA, USA

Benjamin E. Yerys Center for Injury Research and Prevention at CHOP, Philadelphia, PA, USA

Chapter 1
Introduction

Nanette Elster and Kayhan Parsi

> Transition is defined as the movement from adolescence to adulthood in all areas, including home, health care, education, and community. Transition should be a process rather than an event. Optimally, a child, his or her family, and the practitioner should be preparing for transition throughout childhood and adolescence (Shaw 2010).

The prevalence of autism has increased dramatically over the last decade (Maenner et al. 2020). Traditionally, the focus of researchers, policymakers and others has been on autistic children, particularly those children who also have intellectual and developmental disabilities (IDD). However, there is growing interest in the challenges facing autistic young adults. Given that 1 in 54 children are diagnosed as autistic (Maenner et al. 2020), systems must be developed and in place as these children become adults. In fact, a 2020 report by the Centers for Disease Control (Maenner et al. 2020) estimates that there are more than 5,400,000 autistic adults in the United States (Maenner et al. 2020).

The estimate of diagnosed autistic adults is likely understated given that those without IDD during childhood often may not even be diagnosed until adulthood, and, in any event, will continue to increase as more and more children and adults are being diagnosed. This is significant in many respects. One in particular, however, serves as an organizing theme throughout this book—the move from entitlement to eligibility. Children are entitled to services related to being autistic; autistic adults, however, are only eligible for services. The distinction between entitlement and eligibility creates significant legal, ethical and social challenges for autistic adults, as well as for their caregivers and their communities. The shift from entitlement to eligibility has been described by many parents of autistic adolescents as tantamount to "falling off a cliff."

N. Elster (✉) · K. Parsi
Neiswanger Institute for Bioethics, Loyola University Chicago Stritch School of Medicine, 2160 S. First Avenue, Maywood, IL 60153, USA
e-mail: nelster@luc.edu

N. Elster and K. Parsi (eds.), *Transitioning to Adulthood with Autism: Ethical, Legal and Social Issues*, The International Library of Bioethics 91,
https://doi.org/10.1007/978-3-030-91487-5_1

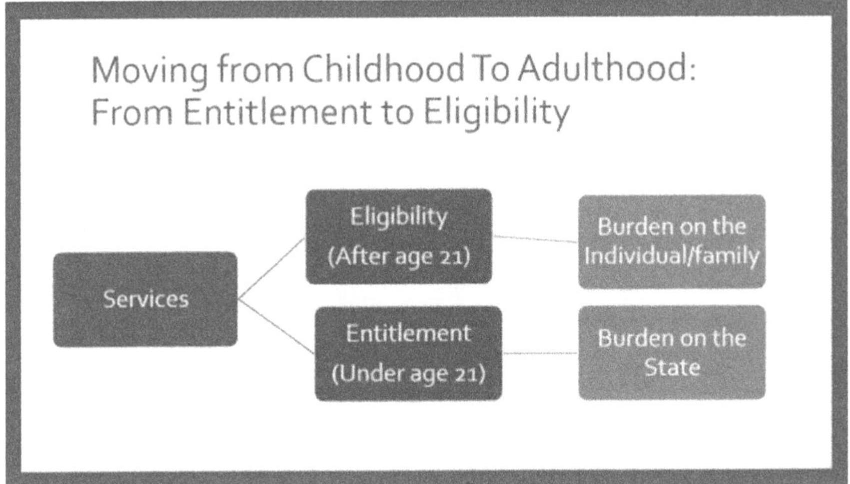

Transition to adulthood is fraught with change and challenge for neurotypical individuals, but for autistic individuals it can mean moving from a range of supports to a seeming abyss with uncoordinated services combined with a host of significant responsibilities.

Although increased attention is being paid to the challenges facing autistic young adults, little coordinated treatment of these myriad issues or set of issues currently exists. The transition to adulthood is marked by many milestones for both the person reaching majority and for their family. Transition itself is a process rather than an event in which one's legal rights and obligations emerge, as does one's ability to exercise and express their autonomy. For instance, the line between dependence and independence becomes increasingly more defined starting around the age of 16, when most adolescents can get a driver's license. Other milestones may include significant life changes, such as going to college or vocational school, obtaining employment, moving into a home of one's own, and managing one's own finances. Other milestones may be more incremental, such as civic participation marked by voting, consuming alcohol, or entering into a romantic relationship which may include marriage and/or reproduction.

This book presents contributions by a variety of authors with expertise on many specific transition markers between childhood and adulthood that may be especially more challenging for autistic individuals than their neurotypical counterparts. While unable to consider every marker of transition, the chapters in this edited volume will focus on: (1) legal and financial management issues, (2) health care issues, (3) reproductive and sexuality issues, (4) educational issues, (5) employment issues, (6) driving and transportation considerations, (7) voting and civic participation, (8) social media/online behaviour issues, and (9) criminal justice issues. The book will conclude with a personal narrative written by an autistic adolescent experiencing many of these transitions. Some chapters are written from an academic, didactic approach whereas others are reflective or descriptive of a particular experience.

The difference in style and tone not only reflects the variability of autism but also enriches the discourse on this complex subject matter (see, NIB). Moreover, the authors address these various issues with the understanding that autism is not a monolithic phenomenon. Some autistic individuals are relatively self-sufficient and require minimal functional support. Others require a significant amount of support and resources. No matter what level of support is needed, a key focus throughout the book is on enhancing and respecting autonomy of the individual and not conflating autonomy and independence. Some authors view autism primarily through a biomedical lens; others through a more holistic lens. These various perspectives reflect the complexity and diversity present within the autistic community.

In Chap. 2, "Legal/Financial Issues Related to Transition," Doyle addresses the different approaches to how decisions are made and deciding who makes those decisions for autistic adults. Such options range from full decision making authority through guardianship or conservatorship to more adaptable approaches such as supported decision making. As we have stated elsewhere, "[t]ransition planning is very individualized. Physical, psychological, and intellectual abilities will all influence how to best support autistic individuals in moving toward adulthood. These same factors will be considered in determining who should make decisions and how" (Elster and Parsi). Doyle examines financial, familial, and feasibility considerations to be considered in determining how to best assist an autistic individual transitioning to adulthood, as well as the longer term implications of such decisions.

In Chap. 3, "Health Care and Transition," Derhammer, Parker, and Rossi-Foulkes discuss the necessary considerations in moving from the pediatric health care environment to the adult health care system. Both the coordination of care and training of health care professionals specific to ASD differ greatly between the pediatric environment where a "medical home" is often the ideal, to the more diffuse adult health care environment. Additionally, if the patient is a minor, parents or guardians are the primary decision makers, but upon reaching majority, the autistic individual has the legal authority to make their own medical decisions (unless a guardian, conservator, or power of attorney is designated). Derhammer and colleagues discuss how medical transition, like transition to adulthood itself, is also a fluid process rather than a singular event.

Chapter 4, "The Taboo Should Be Taught: Supporting Autistic Young Adults in their Sexuality, Intimacy, and Relationships," by Kahn and Kofke, discusses the vast array of topics surrounding reproduction and sexuality for autistic individuals. They consider navigating romantic and sexual relationships, gender and sexuality, consent, and decisions related to reproduction. The World Health Organization (WHO) has long recognized the breadth and importance of sexual health, asserting that "[f]or sexual health to be attained and maintained, the sexual rights of all persons must be respected, protected and fulfilled." Kahn and Kofke present a discussion on how to help empower autistic individuals in making safe and healthy decisions regarding sexuality and intimate relationships.

In Chap. 5, "Transition and Education," Peterson and Strum address requirements for transition planning as well the practical considerations in moving toward post-secondary, vocational or other settings. Many other significant transition markers are impacted by education: where one lives, what kind of job one has, having social connections, etc. In fact, it is at the point when autistic individuals "age out" of the high school setting that the services and supports needed shift from entitlements to the need to apply for and prove eligibility. Peterson and Strum define what transition planning is, why it is important, and explain implementation of a robust transition process employed at *Giant Steps*, an education and therapeutic program for autistic individuals in Lisle, Illinois.

Chapter 6, "Employment issues Related to Transition: Lessons from Aspiritech," Weitzberg presents a model of a successful employment setting (Aspiritech) harnessing the strengths of autistic employees while adapting to their needs. As Roux, et al. have stated: "Employment for wages contributes to individual economic and social well-being, is linked to positive health outcomes, is a gateway to health insurance, and is a factor in quality of life." (Roux et al. 2013). In this chapter, Weitzberg recognizes the enormous contributions that autistic individuals make to the work force while acknowledging the supports that might be necessary to provide benefit to the autistic individual as well as the community.

In Chap. 7, Bishop, Curry, and Yerys discuss "Driving/Transportation and Transition." At age 16 many adolescents will earn their driver's licenses and experience the freedom that comes with that—the ability to drive to school, to work, to visit with friends. The process of earning a driver's license for autistic adolescents is not only challenging, but may be further compounded by other limitations on transportation. Transportation is integral to one's ability to work, to receive healthcare and to socialize with friends, each being important markers for overall well-being and critical to maintaining a certain level of freedom as an adult. A recent scoping review found that clear evidence exists connecting community mobility and driving difficulties to poorer participation and wellness outcomes. Independent community mobility is associated with better employment and education outcomes. Autistic adults and their parents reported that reduced transportation options and lack of mobility skills after leaving school reduced social participation and increased dependence on the parents. (Kersten et al. 2020). Bishop and colleagues focus particularly on the broader significance of driving as well as the barriers to driving faced by autistic individuals.

In Chap. 8, "Autism and Voting Rights," Schnitzler and Yang discuss the importance of civic participation for autistic individuals based on the historic ties between voting rights and disability rights. "Like autism itself, the organizations that purport to represent autistic individuals do not have firm boundaries of representation." (Elster and Parsi 2020). The heterogeneity of the autism community is one of the many reasons why civic engagement is so critical, especially given that many of the support needs of autistic individuals can only be truly addressed with their input. Social engagement, particularly voting, is critical to empowering autistic adults and reflects respect for their autonomy and dignity. Schnitzler and Yang recognize that potential barriers to exercising this right may exist; however, they offer reasons why and potential solutions for how to protect this right.

In Chap. 9, "Autism, the Criminal Justice System, and Transition to Adulthood,"

Richman, Krause-Jensen, and Rodogno take a philosophical and legal approach to analyzing the complexities of how autistic young adults may experience the criminal justice system differently than their neurotypical counterparts. They consider not only how law enforcement officials need to be trained to recognize the potentially confusing or misinterpreted behaviors of autistic individuals, but also how autistic young adults and/or their caregivers must be educated about how to respond to law enforcement. Because the behaviors of autistic individuals may be unfamiliar to law enforcement officers (LEO) this "[l]ack of knowledge of ASD may result in LEOs misinterpreting ASD specific behavior as noncompliant, threatening, disorderly, or suspicious." (Gardner 2019). Richman and colleagues recognize how important clarification and understanding of these behaviors can be, especially as autistic youth move from a juvenile justice system to the adult justice system.

Building upon the potential for misunderstanding of autistic behaviors and intentions in the criminal justice system described in Chap. 9, in Chap. 10, "Social Media/Online Behavior and Transition: A Personal Story of an Attorney Father About His Autistic Son and the Criminal Justice System," Dubin recounts a deeply personal and painful experience his autistic adult son had with the criminal justice system. As a father and lawyer, Dubin candidly shares how his highly educated, rule-following autistic son became entangled in a federal investigation that led to his son being convicted and becoming a registered sex offender. His son Nick's developing sexuality, use of the internet, social limitations/isolation and lack of exposure to/understanding of law enforcement as well as the judicial system's lack of understanding of autism led to such a tragic outcome. Through this painful experience, Dubin offers recommendations to parents, therapists, criminal defense attorneys, prosecutors, and judges about how to better understand and support autistic adults as they navigate the complexities of adult thoughts, feelings and behaviors.

Finally, Chap. 11, "A Personal Perspective on Autism and Transition," by Allanah Elster, describes being a college student and newly identified as neurodiverse. Having an autistic step-brother and being a peer mentor throughout high school to autistic students, Allanah was very familiar with autism, its challenges, and its strengths. She began to realize that she, herself, had been masking her own neurodiversity and therefore sought to be evaluated to better understand herself and her perception of those around her.

The importance of focusing on this transition cannot be overstated. All of the services and assistance provided for autistic children and adolescents will only be meaningful if, as those adolescents become adults, their important contributions to our social fabric can be realized. In his book *NeuroTribes*, Steve Silberman highlights the need to better integrate autistic individuals into our communities. He writes, "instead of investing millions of dollars a year to uncover the causes of autism in the future, we should be helping autistic people and their families live happier, healthier, more productive, and more secure lives in the present" (Silberman 2015). Our hope is that this collection of thoughtful essays will help all of us in our support of the autonomy of autistic individuals during and after their transition into adulthood.

In closing, we would like to acknowledge the many people who made this book possible. First and foremost, we want to thank the contributors of the essays to this collection. Their knowledge, experience and wisdom were indispensable. We also want to thank the editorial staff at Springer, starting with Floor Oosting, who first asked us about ideas for a Springer book. When we mentioned we wanted to edit a book on the ethical, legal and social issues related to transition and autism, she was more than receptive and supportive. We also want to thank the other staff at Springer for their support in getting this book published: Cecil Joselin Simon, Christopher Wilby, Connie Li, and Vidyalakshmi Velmurugan. Their patience with this project is appreciated. We also want to thank the anonymous reviewers who provided their helpful feedback to improve the book. Lastly, we want to thank Loyola University Chicago law student Scott Hulver. He did an extraordinary job in proofreading the manuscript and checking citations. We are indebted to him for his help.

References

Elster, N., and K. Parsi. 2020. Like autism, representation falls on a spectrum. *The American Journal of Bioethics* 20 (4): 4–5.

Gardner, L., Campbell, J.M. and Westdal, J. 2019. Brief Report: Descriptive analysis of law enforcement officers' experiences with and knowledge of autism. *J Autism Dev Disord 49*, 1278–1283. https://doi.org/10.1007/s10803-018-3794-4.

Kersten, M., K. Coxon, H. Lee, and N.J. Wilson. 2020. Independent community mobility and driving experiences of adults on the autism spectrum: A scoping review. *American Journal of Occupational Therapy* 74 (5): 1–17.

Maenner, M.J., K.A. Shaw, J. Baio, et al. 2020. Prevalence of autism spectrum disorder among children aged 8 years—autism and developmental disabilities monitoring network, 11 Sites, United States, 2016. *MMWR Surveillance Summaries 69* (SS-4): 1–12. https://doi.org/10.15585/mmwr.ss6904a1

Roux, et al. 2013. Postsecondary employment experiences among young adults with an autism spectrum disorder. *Journal of the American Academy of Child & Adolescent Psychiatry 52* (9).

Shaw, D. 2010. Transition of adolescents to young adulthood for vulnerable populations. *Pediatrics in Review 31* (12).

Silberman, S. 2015. *Neurotribes: The legacy of autism and the future of neurodiversity*. New York: Avery, Penguin Random House.

Chapter 2
Legal and Financial Issues Related to Transition

Cavan Doyle

Abstract Autistic young adults face unique legal and financial challenges during and after the transition process that may complicate their ability to lead full and productive adult lives. Because many adults with ASD still rely heavily on their families for financial support and assistance in managing many aspects of daily life, this transitional period has important implications for the entire family system. This chapter will examine the important legal and financial implications of the transition to adulthood for individuals with ASD including issues ranging from guardianship of the person to powers of attorney for health care and finance.

2.1 Introduction

Leaving school and transitioning to adulthood presents challenges for adolescents and their families. Turning 18 and becoming a legal adult confers certain rights and responsibilities on all individuals, with or without disabilities. For individuals with Autism Spectrum Disorder (ASD), however, the normative challenges associated with the transition to adulthood are exacerbated by the multiple struggles unique to ASD (Smith et al. 2012). Autistic young adults face unique legal and financial challenges during and after the transition process that may complicate their ability to lead full and productive adult lives. Because many adults with ASD still rely heavily on their families for financial support and assistance in managing many aspects of daily life, this transitional period has important implications for the entire family system.

This chapter will examine the important legal and financial implications of the transition to adulthood for individuals with ASD.

C. Doyle (✉)
AMITA Health, Chicago, IL, USA
e-mail: cavan.doyle@amitahealth.org

N. Elster and K. Parsi (eds.), *Transitioning to Adulthood with Autism: Ethical, Legal and Social Issues*, The International Library of Bioethics 91,
https://doi.org/10.1007/978-3-030-91487-5_2

2.1.1 *Legal Issues*

2.1.1.1 Guardianship

Parents and guardians are the legal decision makers for their children. As soon as a child reaches the age of majority at 18, however, they are legally able to make a number of medical and financial decisions for themselves (including accepting or refusing health care) (Parsi and Elster 2015). For example, parents no longer have the right to insist the child stay in school after the age of 18 if the child does not want to. If a young adult with ASD enters into a contract, the contract is binding—even if they do not fully understand it. Autistic young adults may not be ready to make major life decisions by themselves, and some may never have the skills or capacity to manage complex personal and legal transactions. Although not appropriate in every case, guardianship is one way to protect parents' ability to help their young adult with ASD navigate the adult world. Because guardianship involves considerable restriction of individual rights, it should only be pursued when an autistic young adult is not able to make well-thought out decisions about their own health care and/or choices related to daily life and finances (Rosenblatt and Carbone 2013).

Guardianship is a legally authorized relationship between a competent adult (the guardian) and an incapacitated adult (the ward). It is only possible to gain guardianship of an adult through a legal process that involves a court hearing. There are two types of guardianship (although many parents take on both roles for their young adult child with ASD): (1) guardian of the person, and (2) guardian of the estate. A guardian of the person is responsible for managing the disabled individual's housing, healthcare, and non-medical services such as education and counseling. A guardian of the estate is solely responsible for handling the disabled adult's financial concerns such as managing an estate, property or will.

Guardianship provides parents or guardians with the highest level of continued authority for decision-making on behalf of the autistic adult child and authorizes them to take on legal responsibility for the adult child's daily financial and medical needs. However, depending on the state of residence, the autistic adult may lose a number of legal rights when a guardian is appointed, including, for example, the right to vote and marry. Autistic young adults with lower support needs may operate in a decisional grey zone, in which they have capacity to make some types of decisions but not others. As a result, guardianship should be pursued only in limited circumstances and when it is clear that the individual with ASD is incapable of making considered decisions about major medical and/or financial matters.

2.2 Medical Decision-Making

2.2.1 Health Care Power of Attorney

Despite needing assistance in medical decision-making, some autistic young adults may lack a guardian because they have lower support needs or do not have a parent or family member willing to take on that role (Parsi and Elster 2015). As an alternative to guardianship, a health care power of attorney is a legal mechanism that may allow parents' continued involvement in healthcare decision-making for their autistic young adult children. A health care power of attorney is a document in which the disabled person designates an agent to act as their representative to make decisions about health care in the event the individual is incapacitated or otherwise unable to make those decisions themself. This may be a useful tool when an autistic adult can make some medical decisions but needs help with others.

2.3 Decision-Making Capacity

Adults are presumed to have capacity to make their own health care decisions absent strong evidence to the contrary. There is a specially recognized ethical duty to respect individuals' autonomy with respect to decisions about what does and does not happen to their own bodies (Palmer and Harmell 2016). However, there is also a duty to protect those with diminished capacity for autonomous decision-making (Palmer and Harmell 2016). While a diagnosis of ASD does not automatically mean that a person lacks decision-making capacity, such capacity may wax and wane or vary depending on the specific decision to be made (Parsi and Elster 2015). Health care clinicians must carefully assess the decision-making capacity of autistic adults, with the goal of maximizing individual autonomy while also involving parents and guardians in decisions when appropriate and necessary.

2.4 Sexual Decision-Making and Consent

Experience with individual and partnered sexuality and romantic relationships is common for the majority of autistic adolescents and adults without an intellectual disability (Dewinter et al. 2017). Many autistic individuals may seek sexually intimate experiences and relationships similar to the non-ASD population and demonstrate the entire spectrum of sexual experiences and behaviors (Schöttle et al. 2017). Nevertheless, support for the view of sexuality as a normative part of adult functioning in ASD is relatively recent and contrasts with earlier views that most autistic individuals were asexual or that sexuality was a problematic issue for them (Dewinter et al. 2017).

Several features unique to ASD, such as problems with social interactions and difficulty intuitively understanding non-verbal social cues, may present hidden barriers to the development of healthy romantic and sexual relationships (Schöttle et al. 2017). As a result, "sexuality-related problems can arise, especially at the start of puberty, a time when the development of ASD individuals' social skills cannot keep up with increasing social demands, and the challenges of forming romantic and sexual relationships become particularly apparent" (Schöttle et al. 2017; Seltzer et al. 2003).

The age of legal consent to sexual activity varies from 16 to 18 years of age depending on the state. Although autistic adolescents are generally legally able to consent to sexual activity when they reach these age thresholds, they may face greater challenges than their neurotypical peers as they seek to engage in sexually intimate relationships. In particular, autistic individuals may experience challenges relating to sensory processing issues, having obsessive interests and problems with social and communication skills, leading to relationship difficulties (Turner et al. 2017). They may have difficulty understanding what is involved in different types of sexual activity and may lack the ability to meaningfully consent to such activities. Conversely, challenges in recognizing interpersonal boundaries in social and intimate situations can result in a lack of valid consent by the sexual partners of autistic individuals, which, in some instances, may lead to allegations of sexual assault or rape.

Sex education in adolescence and early adulthood may help address the challenges faced by autistic young adults as they enter into sexual relationships. Unfortunately, some research suggests gaps in the prevalence and usefulness of sex education for this group. In their survey regarding the perception of the adequacy of sex education in a sample of autistic young adults, Hannah and Stagg reported that autistic individuals revealed more difficulties in sexual experience and a lack of educational provisions that adequately met their needs (Hannah and Stagg 2016). Autistic individuals also reported higher levels of social anxiety and noted that they were excluded from peer discussions about sexuality more often (Hannah and Stagg 2016). Finally, they also acknowledged a subjective vulnerability of becoming a victim of sexual abuse, which was not reported by the non-ASD control group (Hannah and Stagg 2016).

Although autistic individuals show an interest in sexual and intimate relationships, they receive less sex education that meets their particular needs (Turner et al. 2017). This deficit may contribute to a decreased ability for autistic individuals to either give valid, legal consent to engaging in sexual activity or seek and receive that consent from a sexual partner. Sexual education programs developed specifically for autistic individuals have become available and may significantly improve sexual knowledge, which in turn could improve sexual experience as part of a healthy and full life (Turner et al. 2017).

2.5 Financial Issues

2.5.1 Shifting from Entitlement to Eligibility

In the public education system, local school systems are the single agency that coordinates educational services for autistic children and adolescents, and special education services are an entitlement for eligible individuals (Revell and Miller 2009). Critically, this single point of service coordination does not exist in adult services, and for the most part, services in the adult system are not entitlement based. Transition-age youth and their families have the potential to receive services and support from a variety of different programs and through several different public and private funding mechanisms. Effective transition from childhood and school to the adult community requires parents or guardians and individuals with ASD to learn about and utilize an array of federal, state and local agencies and organizations.

2.6 Supplemental Security Income (SSI)

Supplemental Security Income (SSI) is an important source of financial support for low-income families raising an autistic child. According to the US Social Security Administration (SSA) there were 1.1 million children under the age of 18 who were receiving SSI in 2019 (SSA 2019c). To qualify for SSI, a child under the age of 18 must have a medically determinable physical or mental impairment or impairments which result in marked and severe functional limitations (SSA 2019c). The impairment(s) must have lasted or can be expected to last for at least one year (SSA 2019c). In a majority of states, being eligible for SSI qualifies a child for the state Medicaid program, which provides access to health care (Rosenblatt and Carbone 2013). The need for affordable health insurance that covers needed services is often what drives families to try to establish SSI eligibility for their children with ASD (Revell and Miller 2009).

SSI is a means-tested program, so there are financial eligibility limitations based on parental income or resources (Revell and Miller 2009). When applying for or receiving SSI, the eligibility and amount of payment for a child SSI recipient below the age of 18 is determined by considering the income and resources of parent(s) responsible for the child SSI recipient's welfare (Virginia Commonwealth University 2017). This process is called "parent-to-child deeming" under SSI program regulations and policies. It is based on the concept that parents who have a responsibility for a child SSI recipient share their income and resources with their child receiving SSI (Virginia Commonwealth University 2017). If deemed parental income and resources exceed the limits set by the SSA, the child is found to be ineligible for SSI and associated Medicaid coverage (Revell and Miller 2009).

SSA handles disability benefits differently for children and adults. When a child recipient of SSI turns 18, SSA reviews their eligibility as if they were applying for the first time, without consideration of previous disability determinations (Revell and Miller 2009). This process is known as the "age-18 redetermination" and catches many families by surprise. Most critically, when a person turns 18, the definition of "disabled" under the SSI program changes, and all SSI recipients are reassessed under the more rigorous adult standard. Individuals who are not determined to be "disabled" under the adult standard may be terminated from SSI cash benefits and lose Medicaid coverage (Revell and Miller 2009).

Establishing SSI eligibility for a young person with ASD is an arduous process that requires a great deal of time, energy and effort. Parents who have waged a long and exhausting battle to establish SSI eligibility may be very reluctant to risk these benefits by having their adolescent pursue paid employment (Revell and Miller 2009). However, there are work incentives built into the SSA that can help those with ASD achieve employment and other goals without risking SSI eligibility. These include the Student Earned Income Exclusion (SEIE) and the Plan to Achieve Self-Support (PASS).

2.7 Student Earned Income Exclusion (SEIE)

As long as a student recipient of SSI remains in school and is younger than 22 years of age, they are able to apply for the Student Earned Income Exclusion (SEIE). SEIE is a special SSI work incentive for young people who are attending school and starting paid employment in preparation for the transition to adult life. In 2019, the SEIE allowed SSI recipients who were younger than 22 and regularly attending school to exclude up to $1,870 of gross earned income a month, up to a maximum annual exclusion of $7,550. (SSA-SEIE 2019d). For the purposes of the SEIE, "regularly attending school" means the student takes one or more courses and attends classes according to one of the following schedules:

- At least 12 h per week in Grades 7 through 12;
- At least 8 h per week in a college or university;
- At least 12 h per week in a training course to prepare for employment (15 h per week if the course involves shop practice); or
- For less time than indicated above for reasons beyond the student's control (e.g. illness) (SSA-SEIE 2019d).

Assuming the student with ASD's monthly gross earnings do not exceed $1,870 per month and $7,550 for the calendar year, they are able to keep the full SSI payment and all of their take-home pay. Further, they could continue to work like this throughout high school without risking SSI payment and Medicaid coverage.

2.8 Plan to Achieve Self-support (PASS)

In addition to the SEIE, another SSI work incentive can be used to help an autistic young adult on the road to gainful employment. A Plan to Achieve Self-Support (PASS) allows a person with a disability to set aside money and assets to pay for items and services needed to achieve a specific work goal (SSA-PASS 2019a). These services include job training or education, support services such as job coaching, job-related items, or virtually anything else needed to achieve an occupational goal (Revell and Miller 2009). Furthermore, income and/or resources set aside in a PASS account do not count when determining SSI eligibility or payments (Revell and Miller 2009). As a result, a student whose income and resources are too high to qualify for SSI may develop a PASS to set aside the excess income and/or resources for their work goal, thus establishing initial SSI eligibility. Alternatively, for someone who has already been found eligible for SSI, a PASS may be used to set aside income or resources that would otherwise cause ineligibility or reduced benefit payments.

2.9 Social Security Disability Insurance (SSDI)

Social Security Disability Insurance (SSDI) is another SSA program potentially available to some adults with ASD. To qualify, an applicant must have a severe mental, psychological, or physical impairment that prevents them from working and must also have sufficient work credits built up over the course of their previous employment. SSDI is an entitlement system available to any disabled person who has paid into the Social Security system for at least ten years, regardless of current income or assets. Unfortunately, many adults, especially young adults, with ASD will not qualify for SSDI because they do not have sufficient work history.

2.10 Medicaid

Medicaid may cover a number of different services for children and young adults with ASD, including services of licensed practitioners, preventive services and therapy services. The scope of these services is defined by each state's particular Medicaid plan and has important financial implications for autistic children and their families. Studies have shown that families living in states with greater per-capita Medicaid coverage experience lower financial costs related to the healthcare of their children with ASD (Parish et al. 2012a, b).

2.11 Home and Community Based Services (HCBS) Medicaid Waiver

The Home and Community Based Services (HCBS) Medicaid waiver is intended to provide services for individuals who, without these services, would need to live in an institutional setting because of the significant nature of their disability. For eligible individuals, the HCBS waiver can provide access to community living and employment (Revell and Miller 2009). Standard services under the HCBS waiver include but are not limited to: case management (i.e. supports and service coordination), homemaker services, home health aides, personal care, adult day health services, habilitation (both day and residential), and respite care.

Although the HCBS waiver can be a resource for autistic individuals who have significant support needs, Medicaid waiver applications are made at the state level and will vary considerably state to state. Transition teams must understand the waiver program in their state in order to appropriately advise autistic young adults and their families about the availability and usefulness of this resource.

2.12 Private Health Insurance

The Affordable Care Act requires health insurance plans and issuers that offer dependent child coverage to make that coverage available until the adult child reaches the age of 26, so autistic children can remain covered by their parents' insurance into their mid-20s. Unfortunately, private health insurance generally does not adequately cover the costs of far-ranging and intense service needs of children with ASD. This gap results in large out of pocket costs for families and can lead to significant financial burden (Friedman et al. 2013). Inadequate private insurance coverage has spurred families to advocate for state parity legislation, which compels private insurers to cover ASD services at levels comparable to other healthcare. As of 2017, 46 states and the District of Columbia had laws mandating insurance coverage for autism services (NCSL 2018). There is promising evidence that families living in states that have adopted private insurance parity mandates experience reduced financial burden related to the healthcare costs of their children with ASD (Parish et al. 2012a, b).

2.13 Employment and Earnings

Employment considerations in the transition to adulthood are covered in-depth in Chap. 5. However, autistic young adults persistently experience underemployment/unemployment at higher rates than their neurotypical peers and often earn lower wages. These factors have important financial implications for both the individual with ASD and their family systems.

2.14 Unemployment/Underemployment

Unemployment and underemployment are enduring problems for individuals with disabilities (Friedman et al. 2013). The Department of Labor estimates that in 2018, just 19% of those with a disability were employed compared to 66% of those without a disability (DOL 2018). The unemployment rate for persons with a disability was 8% in 2018, more than twice the rate of those with no disability (3.7%) (DOL 2018). Furthermore, low employment rates are a constant over the life-course of disabled people (Friedman et al. 2013).

These trends are consistent for employment rates of autistic individuals, who suffer lower rates of both full-time and part-time employment than their neurotypical counterparts (Smith et al. 2012). Taylor and Seltzer found very high rates of unemployment, with only 18% of the surveyed individuals reporting competitive or supported employment (Taylor and Seltzer 2010). Of the young adults in their study who were competitively employed, a large majority were participating in menial, low-paid work and nearly all were working less than 30 hours per week (Taylor and Seltzer 2010). Another study found that after young adults with ASD left the school system, only 6% had competitive jobs and 21% had no employment or educational experiences at all (Shattuck et al. 2012). When they do work, autistic individuals may change jobs frequently, despite (or because of) difficulty adjusting to new job settings. (Müller et al. 2003). Jobs may be poorly paid and often do not provide a living wage (Seltzer et al. 2004). Autistic individuals may also be paid subminimum wage, under a provision of the Fair Labor Standards Act authorizing employers to pay wages that are less than the Federal minimum wage to workers who have disabilities for the work being performed (US Department of Labor). Persistent underemployment and underemployment have clear negative impacts on the lifetime earnings of individuals with ASD, furthering financial strain on family and social support systems. As Ganz noted in his analysis of the lifetime distribution of the costs of autism:

> As [the baby boomers] retire, many of their adult children with autism will be transitioning into adult care settings. Those costs, combined with very limited to non- existent income for their adult children with autism combined with potentially lower levels of savings because of decreased income and benefits while employed, may create a large financial burden affecting not only those families but potentially society in general (Ganz 2007).

2.15 Money Management

Money management may present several challenges to autistic individuals. In particular, two aspects of money management may cause difficulties: (1) understanding the value of money, and (2) handling money appropriately (Smith and Targett 2009).

Autistic individuals may have difficulty understanding the value of money. These challenges will vary from one individual to the next, but may be loosely categorized into three groups. At the first level, a person may not be able to recognize different bills and coins or be able to count or make change. At the second level, an individual can recognize coins and bills but may lack comprehension of the value of money in the marketplace and/or the relationship between work and money. Finally, at a third level, individuals may be able to comprehend the relationship between work and money and have some understanding of what things cost, but still have difficulty with higher levels of money management, such as budgeting and saving.

Poor social skills and difficulty reasoning, both features of ASD, may result in particular challenges in money management. For example, some autistic individuals may hoard money and save every penny that comes their way, which interferes with proper day to day financial self-management and budgeting. Conversely, others may do the opposite, immediately spending money as soon as they have it. Such individuals do not link money with the future; if they have $40 today, they want to spend it today. Transition teams need to be aware of the common pitfalls in the use of money if they are to help autistic young adults learn to manage finances appropriately (Smith and Targett 2009).

Beyond daily finances, credit cards and internet shopping may also give rise to unique challenges for those with ASD. Because e-commerce is less concrete than shopping in a traditional brick and mortar store, autistic individuals may accumulate large amounts of debt with online purchases, without understanding how much money they are spending. Similarly, while young adults with ASD who have low support needs may have access to credit cards, credit use and management is another skill that must be taught and carefully managed in order to avoid accumulation of excessive debt.

2.16 Financial Impacts on Parents and Families

Families provide integral support to autistic young persons as they transition to adulthood. Parents, in particular, continue to be a major source of advocacy and support for people with ASD as they move into adult life (Van Bourgondien et al. 2014). Continued parental involvement into adulthood has important financial impacts on the entire family system.

2.17 Healthcare Costs for ASD Adults

ASD is medically expensive. Autistic individuals incur direct medical expenditures as a result of an elevated need for hospital and emergency services, outpatient, physician and clinic services, medications, behavioral therapy, medical equipment and supplies, and home health services (Smith et al. 2012). Liptak and colleagues reported that the combined healthcare costs of children with ASD were seven times higher than the healthcare costs of nondisabled children (Liptak et al. 2006). These costs continue, and in many cases increase into adulthood, and have long-term financial impacts on families.

2.18 Non-medical Supports and Services

ASD individuals require a multitude of medical, behavioral, therapeutic and educational services, often at a high level of intensity (Smith et al. 2012). The costs of medical and supportive services for children with ASD actually increase as these children enter and transition through adolescence and may persist well into adulthood (Cidav et al. 2013). In investigating cost trajectories of various categories of services among 3–20 year-olds with ASD, Cidav and colleagues found that use of occupational/physical therapy, speech therapy, and diagnostic/assessment services decreased with age, while case management, medication management, day treatment, personal care and respite care increased with age (Cidav et al. 2013). Overall outpatient expenditures increased with age, with much of the increase concentrated in mental health/social skills/behavior modification services, personal care/home health aide services and respite care (Cidav et al. 2013).

2.19 Need for Costly Interventions into Adulthood

Most autistic individuals, including those whose symptoms improve, do not achieve normal functioning in adulthood, and their ASD continues to impair their daily living (Seltzer et al. 2004). The costs of ASD services do not end with childhood, although many of the sources of funding for them do. Because schools are required to provide educational services, they typically pay for a range of ASD therapies, including speech, occupational and physical therapies and behavioral interventions (Friedman et al. 2013). These therapies are expensive, and the need for costly interventions for young people with ASD do not end when they exit the school system, although the schools no longer have an obligation to pay. Studies revealing a positive relationship between increasing child age and rising costs for services as well as a lack of reduction in symptoms as children enter adulthood demonstrate that families are bearing a significant financial burden for their autistic young adult children (Seltzer et al. 2004). In fact, additional lifetime costs for an autistic individual, including medical and non-medical service expenditures, may exceed $3,000,000 (Ganz 2007).

2.20 Housing

Housing often presents one of the greatest challenges for the transition to adulthood for autistic young people. Despite changes in public opinion and social policy about housing for all people with disabilities in recent decades, intended to give autistic individuals and their families more choice in housing options, young adults with ASD continue to live predominantly in the family home (Targett and Smith 2009). Many autistic individuals live at home with their parents well into adulthood. The need to provide living space for an adult child with ASD may prevent parents from reducing their own housing costs (by downsizing into a smaller home, for example) as they age.

2.21 Impact on Parental Earnings and Ability to Work

Having an autistic child has important implications for parents' ability to work and their earnings over the course of a lifespan. Parents' ability to work is often compromised as a result of the demanding, dynamic, and extensive nature of caring for a child with ASD (Smith et al. 2012). Raising an autistic child may influence parents' labor contributions in varying ways. In some instances, parents may increase their work hours to provide health insurance or to pay for costly support services needed by the child with ASD (Cidav et al. 2012). Parents may move from part-time to full-time employment, work overtime, or pursue a second job. These shifts have financial consequences at home, where parents may have to pay for services, including child-care that they themselves previously provided. Increased parental involvement in the workforce in these ways also exacts a social cost of foregone home activities and leisure time (Cidav et al. 2012).

Conversely, parents may reduce their working hours or leave the labor force altogether in order to devote their time to caring for the autistic child. This imposes a cost on the family in the form of lost earnings (Cidav et al. 2012). Families of autistic children may have as much as an average annual loss of 14% of total income (Montes and Halterman 2012). One study reported that family income of families with an autistic child was 28% below that of families of nondisabled children (Cidav et al. 2012).

Cidav and colleagues reported that on average, mothers of autistic children earn 35% less than the mothers of children with another health limitation and 56% less than the mothers of children with no health limitation (Cidav et al. 2012). They are 6% less likely to be employed and work 7 h less per week, on average, than mothers of children with no health limitation (Cidav et al. 2012). High out of pocket expenditures for healthcare and other services, coupled with reduced employment and earnings, increases the probability that having an autistic child creates significant financial burden, including loss of later-life financial security (Sharpe and Baker 2007).

2.22 Financial Planning for Transition

Family financial planning for the autistic young adult child should start well in advance of the child's 18th birthday. An attorney and financial planner specializing in future planning for individuals with special needs can be invaluable to parents in guiding and managing this process. In addition to choosing a guardian or outlining a caregiving succession for their young adult child with ASD, defining who will help make financial and other important life decisions when parents are no longer able to do so, families may utilize several different financial planning instruments.

2.23 ABLE Accounts

One mechanism for providing future financial security for a disabled young adult with ASD is through the establishment of an ABLE account. The Achieving a Better Life Experience (ABLE) Act is a federal law that authorizes states to offer a tax favored account to people with disabilities who became disabled before the age of 26. The money in ABLE accounts can be used for qualified disability related expenses, such as education, housing, health, assistive technology and transportation. Most importantly, ABLE accounts allow people with disabilities to save money without losing eligibility for federally funded benefits such as Medicaid or SSI. In general, there is a $15,000 annual contribution limit and contributions may be made by any "person", including an individual, trust, estate, etc. (National Disability Institute 2019).

2.24 Special Needs Trusts

Another way to provide for financial security into adulthood for autistic individuals is through creation of a Special Needs Trust (SNT). A SNT is a legal tool designed to manage assets for the autistic individual's benefit without compromising eligibility for benefits from governmental programs like Medicaid and SSI (Rosenblatt and Carbone 2013). Money in the SNT can only be used for items and services not covered by Medicaid, SSI or other state or federal funds, and the money cannot be given directly to the autistic person. Instead, it must be given to a third party to pay for goods and services to be used by the disabled individual (Rosenblatt and Carbone 2013).

Parents can establish and fund the trust and act as trustees while they are alive, or the trust can be written so that it is established in the parents' will and starts to function after the parents' death. Any trustee is required to act both in accordance with the provisions of the trust agreement and in the interest of the beneficiary in administering the trust. Because SNTs are subject to state-specific rules and regulations, families should employ the services of an attorney who is familiar with the laws and requirements of their particular state in drafting trust documents.

2.25 Conclusion

The transition to adulthood has important legal and financial implications for autistic young people and their families. Navigating this process can be challenging. Nevertheless, with forethought, advance planning and professional assistance, parents and autistic young adults can mitigate and avoid potential legal and financial pitfalls. Families should start the transition planning process early to give their young adult children with ASD the best possible chance at success, and recognize that financial plans and legal instruments are flexible and may need updating as the young adult ages and their needs evolve.

References

Cidav, Z., S.C. Marcus, and D.S. Mandell. 2012. Implications of childhood autism for parental employment and earnings. *Pediatrics* 129: 617–623.

Cidav, Z., L. Lawer, S.C. Marcus, et al. 2013. Age-related variation in health service use and associated expenditures among children with autism. *Journal of Autism and Developmental Disorders* 43 (4): 924–931.

Department of Labor, Wage and Hour Division. 2018. *Fact Sheet #39: The employment of workers with disabilities at subminimum wages.* https://www.dol.gov/agencies/whd/fact-sheets/39-14c-subminimum-wage. Accessed 30 March 2021.

Department of Labor, Bureau of Labor Statistics. 2021. *Persons with a disability: Labor force characteristics—2021.* https://www.bls.gov/news.release/disabl.nr0.htm. Accessed 20 March 2021.

Dewinter, J., H. De Graaf, and S. Begeer. 2017. Sexual orientation, gender identity, and romantic relationships in adolescents and adults with autism spectrum disorder. *Journal of Autism and Developmental Disorders* 47 (9): 2927–2934.

Friedman, N.D.B., M.E. Warfield, and S.L. Parish. 2013. Transition to adulthood for individuals with autism spectrum disorder: Current issues and future perspectives. *Neuropsychiatry* 3 (2): 181–192.

Ganz, M.L. 2007. The lifetime distribution of the incremental societal costs of autism. *Archives of Pediatrics and Adolescent Medicine* 161: 343–349.

Hannah, L.A., and S.D. Stagg. 2016. Experiences of sex education and sexual awareness in young adults with autism spectrum disorder. *Journal of Autism and Developmental Disorders* 46: 3678–3687.

Liptak, G.S., T. Stuart, and P. Auinger. 2006. Healthcare utilization and expenditures for children with autism: Data from US national samples. *Journal of Autism and Developmental Disorders* 36: 871–879.

Montes, G., and J.S. Halterman. 2012. Association of childhood autism spectrum disorders and loss of family income. *Pediatrics* 121: e821–e826.

Müller, E., A. Schuler, B.A. Burton, et al. 2003. Meeting the vocational support needs of individuals with Asperger syndrome and other autism spectrum disability. *Journal of Vocational Rehabilitation* 18: 163–175.

National Conference of State Legislatures. 2018. *Autism and insurance coverage: State laws.* http://www.ncsl.org/research/health/autism-and-insurance-coverage-state-laws.aspx. Accessed 30 March 2021.

National Disability Institute. *ABLE accounts.* https://www.nationaldisabilityinstitute.org/financial-wellness/able-accounts/. Accessed 30 Sept 2019.

Palmer, B.W., and A.L. Harmell. 2016. Assessment of healthcare decision-making capacity. *Archives of Clinical Neuropsychology* 31 (6): 530–540.

Parish, S.L., K. Thomas, R.A. Rose, et al. 2012a. State insurance parity legislation for autism services and family financial burden. *Intellectual and Developmental Disabilities* 50: 190–198.

Parish, S.L., K. Thomas, R.A. Rose, et al. 2012b. State medicaid spending and financial burden of families raising children with autism. *Intellectual and Developmental Disabilities* 50: 441–451.

Parsi, K., and N. Elster. 2015. A life of one's own: Challenges in the transition from childhood to adulthood with autism spectrum disorder. *AMA Journal of Ethics* 17 (4): 342–347.

Revell, G., and L.A. Miller. 2009. Navigating the world of adult services and benefits planning. In *Autism & the transition to adulthood: Success beyond the classroom*, ed. P. Wehman, M.D. Smith, and C. Schall, 139–162. Brookes, Baltimore.

Rosenblatt, A.I., and P.S. Carbone (eds.). *2013. Autism spectrum disorders: what every parent needs to know*. American Academy of Pediatrics.

Schöttle, D., P. Briken, O. Tüscher, et al. 2017. Sexuality in autism: Hypersexual and paraphilic behavior in women and men with high-functioning autism spectrum disorder. *Dialogues in Clinical Neuroscience* 19 (4): 381–393.

Seltzer, M.M., M.W. Krauss, P.T. Shattuck, et al. 2003. The symptoms of autism spectrum disorders in adolescence and adulthood. *Autism and Developmental Disorders* 33 (6): 565–581.

Seltzer, M.M., P. Shattuck, L. Abeduto, et al. 2004. Trajectory of development in adolescents and adults with autism. *Mental Retardation and Developmental Disabilities Research Reviews* 10: 234–247.

Sharpe, D.L., and D.L. Baker. 2007. Financial issues associated with having a child with autism. *Journal of Family and Economic Issues* 28: 247–264.

Shattuck, P.T., S.C. Narendorf, B. Cooper, et al. 2012. Postsecondary education and employment among young adults with autism spectrum disorder. *Pediatrics* 129: 1042–1049.

Smith, M.D., and P.S. Targett. 2009. Critical life skills. In *Autism & the transition to adulthood: Success beyond the classroom*, ed. P. Wehman, M.D. Smith, and C. Schall, 209–231. Brookes, Baltimore.

Smith, E.S., J.S. Greenberg, and M.R. Mailick. 2012. Adults with autism: Outcomes, family effects, and the multi-family group psychoeducation model. *Current Psychiatry Reports* 14 (6): 732–738.

Social Security Agency. 2019a. *Plan to achieve self-support (PASS)*. https://www.ssa.gov/disabilityresearch/wi/pass.htm. Accessed 17 Sept 2019.

Social Security Agency. 2019b. *Supplemental security income recipients—August 2019*. https://www.ssa.gov/policy/docs/quickfacts/stat_snapshot/#table3. Accessed 17 Sept 2019.

Social Security Agency. 2019c. *Understanding social security income SSI for children*. https://www.ssa.gov/ssi/text-child-ussi.htm. Accessed 17 Sept 2019.

Social Security Agency. 2019d. *Spotlight on student earned income exclusion*. https://www.ssa.gov/ssi/spotlights/spot-student-earned-income.htm. Accessed 17 Sept 2019.

Targett, P.S., and M.D. Smith. 2009. Living in the community. In *Autism & the transition to adulthood: Success beyond the classroom*, ed. P. Wehman, M.D. Smith, and C. Schall, 233–252. Brookes, Baltimore.

Taylor, J.L., and M.M. Seltzer. 2010. Employment and post-secondary educational activities for young adults with autism spectrum disorders during the transition to adulthood. *Journal of Autism and Developmental Disorders* 41: 566–574.

Turner, D., P. Briken, and D. Schöttle. 2017. Autism-spectrum disorders in adolescence and adulthood: Focus on sexuality. *Current Opinion in Psychiatry* 30: 409–416.

Van Bourgondien, M.E., T. Dawkins, and L. Marcus. 2014. Families of adults with autism spectrum disorder. In *Adolescents and adults with autism spectrum disorder*, ed. F. Volkmar, B. Reichow, and J.C. McPartland, 15–40. Springer.

Virginia Commonwealth University. 2017. *Work incentives planning and assistance national training and data center parent-to-child deeming*. https://vcu-ntdc.org/resources/WIPA_OtherResources/ParentToChildDeeming2017.pdf. Accessed 17 Sept 2019.

Chapter 3
Health Care and Transition

Nathan Derhammer, Ellen Parker, and Rita Rossi-Foulkes

Abstract Health Care Transition (HCT) planning is important for all adolescents and is especially crucial for autistic children. Successful transition relies on a general understanding of the transition timeline, which can begin as early as 12 years of age. The transition process is unique for each individual and their family and should be guided by an assessment of readiness. Readiness assessment can be facilitated with the use of a checklist. Health care needs and plans of care can be represented in a portable medical summary to concisely and accurately inform new health care providers. Families of autistic youth can create a Behavior Action Plan for use in unfamiliar environments, including health care encounters. The health care handoff is a fluid process, not an isolated event that relies on constant communication between pediatric and adult health care providers. Resources exist for youth with special health care needs, their caregivers and their health care providers to assist HCT.

3.1 Introduction

Health Care Transition (HCT) planning is important for all adolescents and is especially crucial for autistic children. Adverse outcomes associated with poor HCT include loss of health insurance, discontinuity of care, problems with treatment adherence, patient and family dissatisfaction, higher emergency department utilization, higher hospitalization rates, greater health care costs, and higher unemployment rates. HCT interventions work and have demonstrated improved adherence to care, improved perceived health status, quality of life and self-care skills, increased adult visit attendance, less time between the last pediatric and initial adult visit, decreased hospitalization rates and cost savings (White et al. 2018).

N. Derhammer (✉) · E. Parker
Loyola University Medical Center, 2160 S First Ave, Maywood, IL 60153, USA
e-mail: nderhammer@lumc.edu

R. Rossi-Foulkes
University of Chicago Department of Medicine (Medicine-Pediatrics), Chicago, IL, USA

N. Elster and K. Parsi (eds.), *Transitioning to Adulthood with Autism: Ethical, Legal and Social Issues*, The International Library of Bioethics 91,
https://doi.org/10.1007/978-3-030-91487-5_3

Even for individuals who do not need to transition providers (primary care is provided by Family Medicine or Med-Peds physicians and specialty care is provided by dual-trained specialists), addressing HCT is crucial. Benefits that individuals have received to meet their needs may have age cut-offs. Legal status changes significantly at age 18. Providers, individuals and families will still need to plan for adult health insurance, income supports and disability services if applicable (social security insurance and social security disability insurance), financial planning (creating special needs trusts and ABLE accounts), legal issues (guardianship, durable powers of attorney for health care and / or estate), and autonomy preparedness (see Doyle, Chap. 1). Owing to variations in levels of adaptive functioning, some autistic individuals will be able to make their own HCT plans and others will require lifelong support from their caregivers. To maximize outcomes, the HCT process must be individualized for each person and family.

3.2 The Transition Timeline

Learning Objectives

1. Delineate a typical timeline for the transition process
2. Introduce flexibility and patient-centered variability

The pediatric health care model is characterized by frequent, age-based office visits designed to allow a child and their caregivers to progress through generally predictable developmental and behavioral stages under the guidance of a devoted health care team. From front desk check-in to visit completion, pediatric health care encounters are designed to be supportive and nurturing. Well visits routinely explore growth, sleep, eating habits, social dynamics and academic progress, ending with anticipatory guidance that is often caregiver focused. Sick visits provide patients and their families support and reassurance through times of illness in the safety of a familiar medical home.

Fundamentally, the adult health care model is centered on promoting independent responsibility for lifestyle choices, management of health conditions and the maintenance of health through preventive care interventions. In contrast to the pediatric model, attention shifts from empowering and educating caregivers to a focus on the individual. Patient autonomy is prioritized. Autistic children may not follow the typical progression of development and independent function but are no less deserving of having their personhood respected. Studies suggest that over-estimating independence or failing to identify social and physical barriers to transition can be detrimental to the care of autistic young adults (Anderson et al. 2018).

Without intentional preparation, the transition from the pediatric to the adult health care model can be abrupt and intimidating. This threat applies to both developmentally typical children and those with special needs like autistic children. For this reason, numerous professional societies have developed a transition timeline to facilitate the process. A typical transition timeline, as defined by the "Six Core Elements of Health Care Transition" (AAP Clinical Report November 2018), includes:

(1) Transition policy discussion between ages 12 and 14;
(2) Transition tracking and monitoring between ages 14 and 18;
(3) Transition readiness assessment between ages 14 and 18;
(4) Transition planning between ages 14 and 18;
(5) Transfer and/or integration into adult-centered care between ages 18 and 21; and
(6) Transition completion and ongoing care with adult providers between ages 18 and 26.

Uniformly, the health care transition process begins with a conversation about transition expectations, ideally before adolescence. Pediatric health care practices are encouraged to develop a transition policy that encapsulates their approach to facilitating a step-wise progression to the adult model. Transition policies address the promotion of patient autonomy and independence that is typified by the confidential interview.

The timing of the introduction of confidential interviewing should be both age-driven and developmentally-appropriate. In developmentally typical children, conditionally confidential interviewing—that is, private interviews in which confidentiality will be maintained unless the practitioner identifies a risk of harm to the patient or others—begins around age 13. At the practitioner's discretion and with the support of the patient's caregiver, adolescents with developmental disabilities may begin confidential interviews at a similar or later age. Intellectual disability does and should not preclude confidential interviewing.

As the patient gains confidence and familiarity with confidential interviewing, the practitioner will begin assessing readiness for transition. This assessment could occur informally or through the use of a checklist. In addition to the patient's self-evaluation, caregiver assessment of the patient's readiness for transition should also be assessed.

For individuals with complex health care needs, the transition process represents an opportunity to consolidate the patient's medical history, current management, and future goals of care in a portable medical summary. A portable summary allows the patient and their caregivers to quickly provide insight to health care providers without prior experience caring for the patient in hopes of reducing the risk for unnecessary duplication of prior medical evaluations, avoiding medication errors, and providing more seamless care. This benefit extends to medical specialists, as well.

Transition from pediatric to adult specialty care providers should also be addressed before the child "ages out" of their established specialists. By identifying appropriate adult specialists in early or middle adolescence, both caregivers and health care providers can identify practitioners who are the "right fit" for the patient and are most capable of meeting the young adult's health care needs.

The transition process ends when the young adult has established both general ("primary") care and specialty care with adult health care providers. If the primary care physician changes, a handoff between practitioners is encouraged. Primary care physicians who deliver care to children and adults—namely Family Medicine and Combined Internal Medicine-Pediatrics ("Med-Peds") practitioners—can serve as a source of stability through the transition process and beyond but play an important role in ensuring continuous specialty care.

The remainder of this chapter will explore elements of the health care transition process in greater detail.

3.3 Transition Readiness Assessment

Learning objectives

1. Determine the timing of readiness assessment
2. Define the elements of the transition readiness checklist
3. Compare and contrast assessment of patient and parent/caregiver
4. Utilize the results of a readiness checklist

Assessing readiness for transition serves many purposes. It evaluates the level of insight a young person possesses. It creates awareness of the many components of transition to adulthood, including elements outside what is traditionally viewed as health care. It stimulates important discussions between the health care team, caregivers, and the adolescent themselves.

Active exploration of transition readiness should begin before age 18 but is generally not recommended for individuals younger than 14 years of age. The specific timing of transition readiness assessment should be guided by interest on the part of the adolescent, caregiver insight, and primary care physician judgment. The individual's developmental ability, the complexity of their social and health care needs, and the level of involvement of medical specialists or other ancillary services can all influence the decision to initiate readiness assessment.

The transition readiness checklist offers a concise means of assessing readiness for transition in a variety of domains. Many versions of the transition readiness checklist begin with questions about perceptions of the importance of self-care and confidence in achieving independence. Skills and abilities in the key areas can also be assessed with the following sample questions:

Accessing Health Care

Does the individual speak independently with their physicians?

Do they know their rights with respect to health information privacy?

Can they schedule their physician's visits? Are they able to maintain an updated portable medical summary?

Managing Conditions and Treatments

Can the individual describe their health conditions and disabilities?

Can they list the names and purposes of their medications?

Do they know how to fill prescriptions?

Can they take care of their own medical supplies?

Staying Healthy

Does the individual understand the effect that substance use can have on their condition?

Do they know how their condition affects sexuality?

Do they understand ways to maintain a healthy lifestyle?

Insurance

Can the individual describe what their health insurance covers?

Do they know who to call with questions about insurance?

Do they know how to maintain health insurance coverage?

Other Areas of Transition

Does the individual know resources for adult services, such as transportation?

Do they understand how their condition might affect employment?

Are they aware of any government benefits for which they might be eligible?

Do they know about housing options?

Can they manage their money and pay bills?

Do they understand options for guardianship or power of attorney for health care?

Adolescents, caregivers, and primary care physicians may decide that caregiver-specific checklists are appropriate in certain situations. Checklists designed to be completed by caregivers may be necessary when the adolescent is unable to complete the assessment themselves. Caregiver checklists can also be used to identify alignment or any disconnect between the perceptions of adolescents and those who care for them (Cheak-Zamora et al. 2017).

Readiness assessment checklists and their results can be applied in several ways. First, certain parts of the checklist may be relevant or appropriate at a particular time where other elements may never apply to a given individual. Adolescents, caregivers, and primary care physicians may choose to focus on a specific content area during one clinic visit and defer other areas to future visits. Finally, some or all parts of the checklist can be reassessed at various points along the transition journey.

Assessing readiness—whether through the use of checklists or by other means—creates an important awareness of the multifaceted nature of the transition to adulthood. Open, honest discussion is the most immediate outcome of successful assessment.

3.4 The Portable Medical Summary

Learning objectives

1. Describe the goals of a portable medical summary
2. Define the elements of a portable medical summary

For any number of reasons, children with complex needs may be required to seek health care outside their medical home. One means of organizing health information is referred to as the portable medical summary. As its name suggests, the portable medical summary is a concise and transferrable document.

Maintaining an updated portable medical summary is an important element in the transition to adulthood. A strong working knowledge of the components of a portable medical summary empowers an individual to represent themselves, their conditions, and their needs in new or unfamiliar health care settings.

The portable medical summary goes beyond simply representing medical conditions and their treatments. Suggested elements are defined as follows (adapted from the Got Transition® Six Core Elements of Health Care Transition™ 3.0 Sample Medical Summary and Emergency Care Plan (White et al. 2020):

Contact Information

In addition to the patient's name, nickname and preferred language, parent/caregiver information should be included, along with the best time and mode of communication.

Emergency Care Plan

This section quickly identifies common emergent presenting problems, suggested tests and treatment considerations. Emergency contact information can also be listed.

Allergies and Procedures to be Avoided

Many health care providers are familiar with obtaining allergy information as it pertains to medications and environmental exposures, including dietary restrictions. For youth with special health care needs, delineating procedures and medications to avoid, along with explanations, may reduce unnecessary and potentially distressing interventions for patients and their caregivers.

Diagnoses and Current Problems

An inclusive list of medical diagnoses, as well as active problems in a broad range of domains (behavioral, feeding and swallowing, learning, physical anomalies, sensory, etc.) creates an awareness of the array of medical needs, therapy services and social/academic accommodations an individual may require.

Medications

Prescription and over-the-counter medications, as well as herbal supplements, should be included to alert health care providers to potential adverse effects and drug interactions.

Health Care Providers

Youth with special health care needs often receive multidisciplinary services. In addition to physicians and advanced practice providers, therapists, counselors and case managers can be included in the list.

Prior Surgeries, Procedures, and Hospitalizations

Knowledge of prior surgeries and procedures informs medical decision-making. Patterns of hospitalization, as well as summaries of particularly complicated or prolonged hospital stays, are especially informative.

Baseline Status

In any given health care encounter, understanding a patient's baseline vital signs—namely temperature, blood pressure, heart rate, and respiratory rate—allows a health care provider to objectively assess any deviation from normal in an individualized way. Baseline neurological status, including level of interaction with caregivers and the environment, is equally important. Delineating baseline abnormal physical findings (weakness or position of an arm or leg, breathing sounds, etc.) and lab results (kidney function, blood counts, etc.) puts current findings in a patient-centered context.

Most Recent Labs and Radiology

Radiographic images (chest X-rays, MRI studies, etc.) and detailed reports of various studies (electroencephalogram or EEG, electrocardiogram or EKG, biopsy results, etc.) may not be immediately available to a health care provider. A short summary is typically sufficient while awaiting detailed medical records.

Equipment, Appliances, and Assistive Technology

Youth with special health care needs may rely on alternative means of feedings, such as a gastrostomy tube, respiratory support or a communication device, among other technology. Listing physical appliances, like crutches, orthotics, or a walker, can be especially useful for rehabilitation specialists.

School and Community Information

Agency and school personnel may require updated information on changes in functional status or new needs, whether temporary or permanent.

Portable medical summaries are living, breathing documents. Regular review and updating is essential. Including the most recent date of revision quickly informs any reader how current the information contained may be. While the information contained in a typical summary is helpful, autistic youth may benefit from a uniquely designed plan for behavior management, what these authors will refer to as a Behavior Action Plan.

3.5 Autism Management Plan

Objectives

1. Review medical conditions that can lead to behavior dysregulation
2. Review conditions in the delivery of medical care that can trigger behavioral decompensation: inpatient, Outpatient and Telehealth Environments
3. Assess individual behavior scripts
4. Develop a Behavior Action Plan.

Many conditions can lead to behavior dysregulation in autistic children. Common childhood medical conditions or developmental processes such as ear infections, constipation and menstruation can lead to physical symptomatology and internal stimuli that are challenging to express and emotionally interpret (Autism Speaks 2017). More acute medical conditions, like appendicitis, not only lead to intrinsic behavior challenges but also require children to seek medical care in an environment that often increases anxiety. Autistic children are at risk for many of the same childhood ailments as their peers. However, due to communication differences they may not be able to describe their presenting symptoms in a way that readily identifies the cause to their physician. Often their presenting symptom or behavior change is common to many diagnoses and this may lead to extra, sometimes invasive, tests to confirm a suspected diagnosis which, in part, leads to additional healthcare anxiety (Table 3.1).

The health care environment itself is frequently very challenging for autistic children to navigate because of copious, unfamiliar sensory stimuli that are overwhelming: flashing glowing lights, loud beeping monitors, physical touch from strangers, and confining unfamiliar exam rooms (Table 3.2).

Until very recently, most families were required to physically bring their child into a medical facility to receive care. In March 2020 with the advent of COVID-19, the Centers for Medicare and Medicaid Services (CMS) lifted restrictions on telehealth services and, for the first time ever, patients everywhere were able to access medical services from home for both COVID and non-COVID ailments (Center for Medicare and Medicaid 2020). The advent of telehealth has since revolutionized patient access by decreasing barriers to care that existed even before COVID: transportation, physical mobility, and sensory dysregulation.

Telehealth has been particularly helpful in providing access to autistic children by allowing them to remain in a familiar environment during their visit. However, telehealth also comes with very distinct challenges for this patient population, medical providers, and caregivers alike. Telehealth requires reliable network connections and devices to allow synchronous audio and video visits, for which patients and caregivers may not have access. And while audio-only telephone visits are allowed by CMS, the inability to visually inspect or examine a patient's demeanor, general appearance, and response to interventions substantially limits the diagnostic power of the clinician. A comprehensive physical exam to inspect the ears or abdomen for example, is limited in this modality and may ultimately result in a second in-person

Table 3.1 Common childhood illnesses and behavior implications

	Common childhood ailments	Behavior implications
Infectious diseases	Viral illness, UTI, Skin Infection, Ear Infection, Sinus infections, Dental Infection, Pneumonia, Appendicitis	Pain, Irritability, Fatigue
Head & neck disorders	Sore Throat, Ear Ache, Laryngitis, Impairment of Sensory Organs: Vision, Hearing, Taste, or Smell	Pain, Disorientation, Impaired Language
Gastrointestinal & nutritional disorders	Constipation, Diarrhea, Bloating, Reflux, Gastritis, Nausea, Malnutrition, Obesity, Swallowing Disorders	Pain, Irritability, Fatigue, Poor Growth and Concentration
Nervous system disorders	Headaches, Seizure disorders	Pain, Impaired Concentration, Confusion, Fatigue
Musculoskeletal disorders	Joint Sprains, Fractures, Bruises	Pain, Irritability, Mobility Restrictions
Psychiatric disorders	Insomnia, Generalized Anxiety, Major Depression, ADHD, OCD	Impaired Concentration, Stress, Anxiety, Fatigue, Irritability
Sexual organ disorders	Menstrual Cramps and Excessive Bleeding, Ovarian cysts	Pain, Irritability, Fatigue, Nausea and Appetite disturbances
Hematologic disorders	Anemia	Fatigue, Irritability
Pharmacologic disorders	Accidental and Non-Accidental Ingestions, Medication Side Effects	Sleepiness, Fatigue, Irritability, Impaired Concentration

Table 3.2 Environments of care

	Outpatient	Inpatient	Telehealth
Challenges	Confined space	Multiple New Providers	Limited Physical Exam
	Physical touch	Invasive Treatments	Can't complete testing
	Some Invasive Tests	New environment, Bright lights, Noises	Technical glitches
Benefits	Familiar Doctor	Coordinate services	Home Environment
	Access to diagnostic testing	Access to higher level of care	No transportation needed

office visit to confirm a diagnosis based on physical exam findings or laboratory tests. Nonetheless, telehealth encounters serve as a good first step in health care evaluation, providing in home physician assessments and reducing external stimuli associated with doctor's offices.

Over time, many families who access in-office medical care overcome the sensory struggles by developing a planned routine with a trusted (often pediatric) caregiver with whom their child becomes familiar. Maintaining consistency in the same clinical environment with the same health care providers becomes paramount to avoiding behavioral dysregulation. However, as children approach adulthood, it becomes necessary to discuss transitioning them to adult health care providers, often in an adult health care model that is unfamiliar to both the young adult and family.

The health care transition can be anxiety-producing for everyone and fear of behavioral dysregulation in a new environment can be all-consuming. However, simply reflecting on the successes or failures of prior experiences can aid in creating a toolbox of skills to anticipate and address behavioral decompensation during the impending health care transition. Many families already have their toolbox packed without even knowing it because, as parents, they are experts in their child's behavior script (Bearss et al. 2018). Behavior scripts are repeated behaviors or actions that are predictable or stereotypical for an individual, such as consistently crying whenever loud music is played or relaxing with the application of a weighted blanket. Each behavior is specific to the individual child. Caregivers, including teachers, often know these behavior scripts well and consciously or unconsciously avoid actions that will cause disruptive behavior and engage in positive acts that will elicit calming behaviors (Dunlap and Dyer 2016).

Health care providers may not be experts in the behavior scripts of an individual child, particularly if it is the first time they are providing care for that individual. It is therefore important that parents educate healthcare providers about their child, not just their medical conditions but also their behavior scripts. Through shared communication about these behaviors, anxiety can be decreased for the caregiver, child and health provider alike.

Given the time constraints that often exist with health care encounters, it is best to plan ahead and define on paper some of the child's specific behavior scripts. Creating such a document—a Behavior Action Plan—will allow the caregiver to reflect on both aggravating and alleviating actions and concretely document them in a form that can be shared with any health care provider, teacher or future caregiver. Below is an example of a completed Behavior Action Plan (Fig. 3.1):

When constructing a Behavior Action Plan, patient factors should be listed first. It is important to reflect on all environments where behavior is observed: home, school, after school programs, work, etc. Different behaviors and soothing responses are elicited with different people and places and all should be included. If caregivers have had prior health care experiences and know what factors specifically caused conflict, then those factors should be listed individually under Medical Environment.

As they develop the Toolbox section, caregivers should reflect on all things that help soothe. These include physical objects of comfort and actions or behaviors that bring joy, as well as necessary requests from others to avoid or modify their

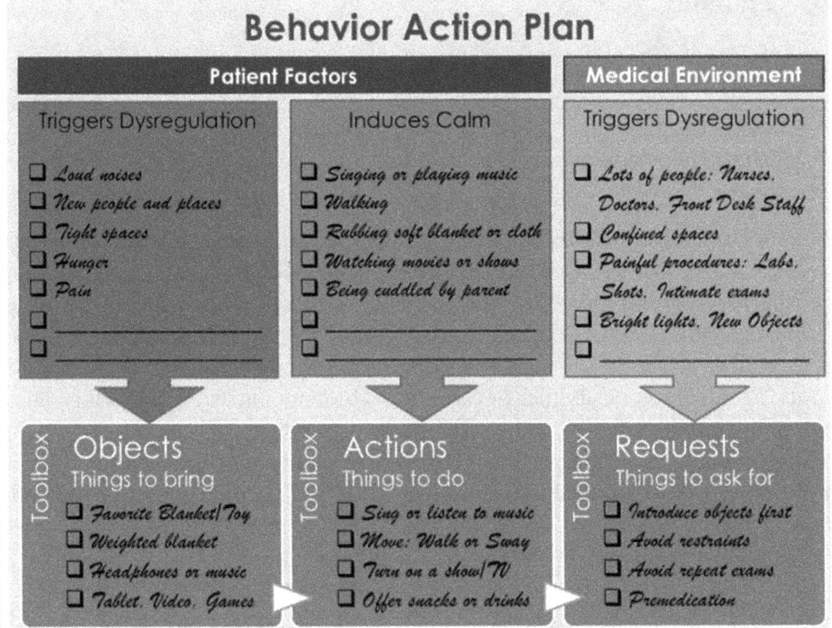

Fig. 3.1 Sample behavior action plan

behavior when caring for the child. In medicine, procedures themselves, like inserting a needle to draw blood, may not be modifiable but the approach taken certainly can be. Caregivers should feel empowered to collaborate with health care providers to identify modifications that may be less anxiety-producing.

After completing a Behavior Action Plan, the initial goal is for the document to be reviewed at routine health visits with an established pediatric provider to elicit input and practice the Toolbox techniques in a familiar environment. The Behavior Action Plan should be updated as the child grows, as behaviors change, and as new health care encounters reveal additional successful techniques. When the time for transition arrives, the Behavior Action Plan can be shared with adult providers knowing that it has already been successfully utilized. The Toolbox should also guide medical subspecialist visits, dental appointments, psychiatric care and unplanned acute care visits to the ER or urgent care. Collaboratively combining caregiver knowledge of the behavior scripts of a young autistic adult with a medical professional's knowledge of health care interventions can contribute to minimizing behavioral conflicts during transition.

3.6 Handoff

Objectives

1. Review the individualized nature of the handoff timeline
2. Define the handoff and set expectations for all involved parties

The culmination of all transition planning and preparation is the health care handoff. Rather than a discrete moment in time or singular event, the handoff is a fluid process. In anticipation of health care transition, pediatric providers of both primary and specialty care should deliver the results of readiness assessment, a copy of the portable medical summary and an updated Behavior Action Plan to adult providers. In turn, adult providers should acknowledge and review the content of these documents. Residual responsibilities of care should be communicated between pediatric and adult care providers to address the needs of the medical plan of care moving forward (White and Schmidt 2020). Direct communication between providers is encouraged and ideally occurs before the initial adult provider visit to help plan for accommodating special needs. Pre-visit planning allows for decreased anxiety amongst all parties.

The initial adult visit should not be seen as the "transfer of care" visit but instead as an opportunity to assess rightness of fit. Transferring care is a high stakes endeavor and can be an emotionally charged experience for all parties. The visit itself should be an opportunity to review transfer documents and address any concerns the young adult and their family may have about transitioning to the adult model of care. Important issues to address at this visit include setting expectations for methods of communication, shared decision making and information access (White and Schmidt 2020). Access to pediatric providers should not cease after the initial encounter with adult providers. Pediatric providers should remain available for medication reconciliation, refills, coordination of care and acute care visits as necessary even after the initial adult visit to avoid a sense of abandonment. However, young adults should be encouraged to seek advice and consultation from their new adult providers to strengthen their skills in navigating the adult health care system.

Transfer completion is dependent on a number of factors but relies heavily on readiness assessment to determine the degree of skill acquisition and comfort the young adult has with the adult care model. Constant feedback and encouragement is needed from both pediatric and adult providers to assess when the handoff can be deemed complete. Direct contact is again encouraged between pediatric and adult care providers to allow for closed loop communication and to avoid ambiguity which often leads to increased anxiety. The timeline for the handoff is patient and provider specific and should be a dynamic process that adjusts to feedback.

It is possible that a chosen adult provider may not be considered a good fit for the young adult or family. The handoff plan (and pediatric providers themselves) must be flexible enough to allow for identification of an alternative adult provider. Families should be counseled about this "rightness of fit" when searching for an adult medical home and advised not to be discouraged should the initial handoff be unsuccessful

(White and Cooley 2018). The act of transition should not be abandoned but re-evaluated in its approach. Ultimately, the goal is to build a collaborative partnership between the young adult and their adult health care provider. Achieving this goal takes thoughtful planning and willingness from all parties.

3.7 Resources and Putting It All Together

Learning objectives

1. Recognize areas of the transition process requiring additional resources
2. Provide examples of resources, teaching, and toolkits to address the above areas
3. Illustrate an example of the transition process

Utilizing resources for transition can help patients, families and health care providers develop HCT plans that serve their individualized needs. Autism Speaks has a transition toolkit that can be downloaded and includes all aspects of transition, including several aspects of health care including finding the right doctor, mental health, personal hygiene, and puberty/sexuality (Autism Speaks 2020). The American Academy of Pediatrics developed a toolkit outlining a process called STEPS (below), for providers to use to support adolescents with autism spectrum disorder and their parents through the HCT process (American Academy of Pediatrics 2019a, b):

> **S**tart the HCT process early, typically when the adolescent is between 12 and 14 years of age, and give the adolescent and family time to prepare mentally for leaving the pediatric practice.
>
> **T**alk with parents about their role in the transition process by explaining how they will move from a leadership role in managing their child's health care to a supporting role. Parents and providers should also talk with the adolescent to encourage them to be engaged in decision-making.
>
> **E**ducate the adolescent and parents about his or her health condition and encourage the adolescent to ask questions
>
> **P**artner with the adolescent and family in identifying adult health care professional(s).
>
> **S**upport the adolescent and family through the process by preparing a transfer of care letter and portable health summary, scheduling time to consult with the transitioning provider, and providing emotional support.

Practical tools are publicly available for every part of the HCT process. Starting at age 12–14, providers should discuss HCT and the medical practice's policy regarding HCT. Adolescents and their caregivers should complete HCT readiness assessments and set HCT goals at least annually. Got Transition, a cooperative agreement between the Maternal and Child Health Bureau and the National Alliance to Advance Adolescent Health, provides several tools for HCT including sample practice policies, HCT timelines, individualized HCT flow sheets, HCT readiness assessments, portable medical summaries and emergency plans of care (Got Transition2020). The American College of Physicians Pediatric to Adult Care Transitions Initiative provides similar tools that are specific to an adolescent or young adult's condition (American College of Physicians 2019). In addition, Good 2 Go Transition Program provides a tool, "My Health Passport," a customized, wallet-sized card that provides instant access to an individual's medical information (Kaufman 2012). The Autistic Self Advocacy Network (ASAN) is a non-profit organization run for and by autistic people. ASAN's publication, "*Transition to Adulthood: A Health Care Guide for Youth and Families,*" provides information about obtaining adult health insurance and income supports, information about guardianship versus supportive decision making, durable powers of attorney for health care, and HCT planning through school (Autistic Self Advocacy Network 2012). The AASPIRE worksheet enables individuals to learn how to prepare for and schedule an appointment with a health care provider, what to bring to the visit, how to describe symptoms, how to get help after the visit and how to carry out various aspects of the health care plan including getting medical tests, scheduling with specialists and following up with the provider (Academic Autistic Spectrum Partnership in Research and Education 2020). Individuals, caregivers, and health care providers can publicly access these tools to aide in the transition process.

Putting it all together

AB is a 14-year-old autistic girl. She enjoys painting and horseback riding. She also has asthma and has recently developed seizures. Her parents manage all aspects of her care including scheduling doctor's appointments and ordering her prescription medications. They have worked closely with her pediatrician, neurologist and pulmonologist to coordinate her treatments by using her personalized Behavior Action Plan. This has worked very well to help her when she needs invasive testing such as blood draws and nebulizer treatment for her asthma. She also uses picture cues at school and for medical procedures to help her learn new tasks and adjust to changes in her schedule.

AB's pediatrician informed AB and her parents their practice's policy regarding HCT. Starting now, each year, AB will have a HCT visit. At each visit, both AB and her parents will complete a HCT readiness assessment checklist to identify specific HCT goals for the coming year. The pediatrician, with the help of AB and her parents, will also create a portable health summary and be sure it is updated each year. AB and her parents complete "My Health Passport" to aid in completing the portable health summary. All health care providers, AB and her parents will have a copy of these important documents. AB's parents also learn about special needs trusts and health care savings plans that may help them plan for AB's future health care needs. Additionally, the pediatrician addresses with AB and her parents issues around hygiene, puberty and sexuality. By age 16, AB will spend some time alone with the pediatrician to practice communicating her needs to health providers. By age 22, AB will be fully transferred to adult health care primary and specialty care providers. AB and her parents are nervous about the prospect of leaving the pediatrician's practice. The pediatrician assures AB and her parents that AB will not be transferred without extensive preparation.

Each year, AB and her parents, along with the pediatrician, identify a specific HCT goal and identify specific tools they can use to achieve this goal. By age 16, the pediatrician's office provides AB and her parents with information about applying for adult health insurance, disability services, and income supports and the timeline needed to assure that AB will not have gaps in care or support (see Doyle, Chap. 1). The pediatrician and AB's parents explore the need for adult guardianship versus other forms of supportive decision making such as durable powers of attorney for health care. They also start to explore adult health care providers including neurologists, pulmonologists and primary care providers (see Doyle, Chap. 1).

At age 17, AB and her parents select adult health care providers and schedule a visit with each. In advance of the visit, the pediatrician sends the portable health summary to the providers and includes in the summary skills that AB can master on her own and skills she needs her parents to navigate. Because AB has been admitted to the pediatric hospital about once per year for her asthma, she and her parents also take a "field trip" to the adult hospital. After AB attends these adult health care appointments, she and her parents discuss with the pediatrician how each visit went and if modifications need to occur regarding the choice of adult health care providers.

At age 18, AB signs a release giving permission for all providers to discuss issues surrounding health care with her parents as she is able to make decisions and personally perform several actions regarding her health care but needs her parents' input to help her. AB's parents become her durable power of attorney for health care.

At age 19, by using picture cues, AB has learned to use the patient portal for her electronic medical record. She has learned how to schedule her own doctor appointments and request refills for her prescriptions. She and her parents have identified a different adult pulmonologist, as she was uncomfortable with the original pulmonologist's appointment. AB again sees the adult primary care provider and neurologist she met the prior year. They are impressed that she has learned additional skills for her health care.

At age 20, AB and her parents request to be transferred to all adult health care providers as it is now more convenient for them as they are all in the same practice group and building. AB, her parents and the pediatrician update AB's portable health summary and send it to all her providers.

AB's HCT is a success story. Her pediatrician started the process early, clearly communicating the practice's policy and the steps involved in the transition process to AB and her family. AB achieved supported autonomy, tailored to her individual abilities and wishes. She did not suffer a gap in health insurance coverage or access to her health care team and was able to plan for her future financial needs and supportive services. Throughout the HCT process, AB's pediatrician provided AB and her family with information and tools addressing all aspects of HCT ensuring that they were fully informed and supported.

Achieving a successful HCT requires a partnership between individuals, their families, care givers, and members of the health care team. There is a wealth of publicly available tools to assist all members of the team in navigating this critical process. Key aspects in the HCT process include starting the process early and clearly communicating the practice's HCT policy, timeline, and process. Scheduling regular visits devoted to HCT at least annually throughout the process provides all members of the team a chance to evaluate unmet needs and outline the next steps. A successful HCT is crucial to maximize health and ability for autistic individuals.

References

Academic Autistic Spectrum Partnership in Research and Education. 2020. Healthcare toolkit for patients & supporters: Forms & worksheets. https://autismandhealth.org/?a=pt&p=main&t=pt_frm&theme=ltlc&size=small. Accessed 6 Nov 2020.

American Academy of Pediatrics. 2019a. *Autism—caring for children with autism spectrum disorders: a practical resource toolkit for clinicians*, 3rd edn. Itasca: American Academy of Pediatrics.

American Academy of Pediatrics. 2019b. Ten common childhood illnesses and their treatments. https://www.healthychildren.org/English/health-issues/conditions/treatments/Pages/10-Common-Childhood-Illnesses-and-Their-Treatments.aspx. Accessed 14 Oct 2020.

American College of Physicians. 2019. ACP pediatric to adult care transitions initiative: Condition specific tools. https://www.acponline.org/clinical-information/high-value-care/resources-for-clinicians/pediatric-to-adult-care-transitions-initiative/condition-specific-tools. Accessed 6 Nov 2020.

Anderson, K.A., C. Sosnowy et al. 2018. Transition of individuals with autism to adulthood: a review of qualitative studies. *Pediatrics* 141(s4). https://doi.org/10.1542/peds.2016-4300I

Autism Speaks. 2017. Autism and health: a special report by Autism Speaks. Advances in understanding and treating the health conditions that frequently accompany autism. https://www.autismspeaks.org/science-news/autism-and-health-special-report-autism-speaks. Accessed 14 Oct 2020.

Autism Speaks. 2020. Transition tool kit. https://www.autismspeaks.org/tool-kit/transition-tool-kit. Accessed 6 Nov 2020.

Autistic Self Advocacy Network. 2012. Healthcare transition toolkit: Transition to adulthood: a health care guide for youth and families. https://autisticadvocacy.org/wp-content/uploads/2014/07/ASAN-healthcare-toolkit-final.pdf. Accessed 6 Nov 2020.

Bearss, K., C. Johnson, et al. 2018. *Parent training for disruptive behavior: The RUBI autism network, parent workbook*. New York: Oxford University Press.

Center for Medicare and Medicaid. 2020. Medicare telemedicine health care provider fact sheet. https://www.cms.gov/newsroom/fact-sheets/medicare-telemedicine-health-care-provider-fact-sheet. Accessed 14 Oct 2020.

Cheak-Zamora, N.C., M. Teti, et al. 2017. Exploration and comparison of adolescents with autism spectrum disorder and their caregiver's perspectives on transitioning to adult health care and adulthood. *J Pediatric Psych.* 42 (9): 1028–1039.

Dunlap, K., S. Dyer. 2016. Behavioral response script development guide. https://www.apbs.org/sites/default/files/conference-2016/presentations/j9-behavior_response_script_development_guide-apbs2016.pdf. Accessed 6 Nov 2020.

Got Transition. 2020. Resources & Research. https://www.gottransition.org/resources-and-research/. Accessed 6 Nov 2020.

Kaufman, M. 2012. Good 2 go transition program: MyHealth passport. https://www.sickkids.ca/myhealthpassport/. Accessed 6 Nov 2020.

White, P.H., A. Schmidt. 2020. Six Core Elements: Integrating young adults into adult health care package. https://www.gottransition.org/6ce/?integrating-full-package. Accessed 1 Oct 2020.

White, P.H., W.C. Cooley et al. 2018. Supporting the health care transition from adolescence to adulthood in the medical home. *Pediatrics* 142(5). https://doi.org/10.1542/peds.2018-2587

White, P.H., A. Schmidt et al. 2020. Sample medical summary and emergency plan of care. In *Six Core Elements: transitioning youth to an adult health care clinician. Got Transition 3.0.* https://gottransition.org/6ce/?leaving-full-package. Accessed 6 Nov 2020.

Chapter 4
The Taboo Should Be Taught: Supporting Autistic Young Adults in Their Sexuality, Intimacy, and Relationships

Laurie Gutmann Kahn and Marisa Kofke

Abstract This chapter provides a foundation for supporting and empowering autistic youth and young adults to make healthy and safe decisions about sexuality and relationships during the transition to adulthood. One chapter cannot cover all of the barriers and strategies concerning dating, intimacy, and sexuality for everyone's individual needs. Instead, this chapter is designed to explore a way of thinking about talking about sex and sexuality to support autistic young adults. The topics covered include sexuality and intimacy (including consent, masturbation, and self-advocacy), relationships (flirting, dating, stalking and abuse), gender and sexuality identity (LGBTQ+ identity, gender identity), sexuality education, and concludes with implications for transition (marriage, partnership, reproduction, raising children, and family).

4.1 Introduction

> Sexuality is often the source of our deepest oppression; it is also often the source of our deepest pain. It's easier for us to talk about -and formulate strategies for changing - discrimination in employment, education, and housing than to talk about our exclusion from sexuality and reproduction (Finger 1992, p. 9).

4.2 Sexuality, Autism, and Transition

This chapter provides a foundation for supporting and empowering autistic youth and young adults to make healthy and safe decisions about sexuality and relationships during the transition to adulthood. One chapter cannot cover all of the barriers and strategies concerning dating, intimacy, and sexuality for everyone's individual needs.

L. G. Kahn (✉) · M. Kofke
Moravian College, 1200 Main Street, Bethlehem, PA 18017, USA
e-mail: kahnl@moravian.edu

N. Elster and K. Parsi (eds.), *Transitioning to Adulthood with Autism: Ethical, Legal and Social Issues*, The International Library of Bioethics 91,
https://doi.org/10.1007/978-3-030-91487-5_4

Instead, this chapter is designed to explore a way of thinking about talking about sex and sexuality to support autistic young adults. We know that parents and teachers may not feel adequately prepared to have supportive conversations around sex and sexuality (Holmes et al. 2016; Mehzabin and Stokes 2011). Also, students with disabilities have limited access to the "ignored curriculum" or the important social knowledge acquired through peers to learn norms and behaviors toward sex and sexuality (Gougeon 2009). It is clear that absence of the ignored curriculum and information from parents and teachers significantly affects autistic young adults' access to full citizenship, (Gougeon 2009) and quality of life as they transition to adulthood.

For all children, the family background and home environment impact the development of personal boundaries, relationships, and social norms. Cultural and religious beliefs influence approaches to children's sexual development. Parents are often the first source of information when it comes to sexuality, so when there are omissions in communication, young adults likely gain their information from unreliable—and possibly unsafe or ableist—sources (Mehzabin and Stokes 2011). As reported by Holmes et al. (2016), the majority of parents of autistic adolescents discuss privacy with their children, including private body parts, bodily functions including reproduction, masturbation (where appropriate), good touch/bad touch and reporting unwanted touching. Yet few reviewed consent, dating, love, romantic rejection, birth control, STDs, sexual slang, masturbation, sexual activities, etc. If parents view their children as "low functioning," they are less likely to explicitly discuss relationships, sexual health, and the prevention of unwanted behaviors and outcomes.

There is a significant need for increasing training and guidance for educators. Students with IEPs and modified diplomas are often left out of sexuality education courses, if they are offered in schools at all. Special educators and inclusive teachers are not given enough training in sexuality and relationship education. Health educators are also not adequately trained to educate diverse learners (Curtiss and Ebata 2016). As allies (family, friends, professionals, etc.), we must critically comprehend our own biases, values, and knowledge limitations around sexuality, relationships, and health, so autistic young adults can be provided with meaningful and individualized guidance and education. This chapter purports to engage in a strength-based discussion of the barriers that autistic people face regarding sexual health, sexuality, intimacy, relationships, and family planning, as well as explores ways non-autistic allies can support them during the transition to adulthood. This is a topic often left out of the larger discussion on transition for young adults with disabilities. As the World Health Organization (WHO) recognizes how important sexual health and sexual activity are to overall health (WHO 2006, updated 2010), we believe this topic is necessary for the overarching goal of achieving a high quality of life for autistic adults.

4.3 Theoretical Framework

Before we continue to explore specific phenomena and research concerning sexuality and autistic young adults, we want to explain the lens that we are utilizing to understand the issues and provide future directions. We approach this work using a social model of disability framework influenced by a neurodiversity perspective.

Positionality. As teachers, researchers, and disability activists, our positionalities shape the lens in which we view this information. Our identities, experiences, and values determine our theoretical framework, the information we choose to present, and the voices whom we illuminate. In stating our positionalities, we acknowledge our privileged positions as highly-educated, heterosexual, white, cisgender women with non-disabled children, who are Jewish (Dr. Kahn) or grew up Catholic (Dr. Kofke) as well as the experiences that led us to understand autism, transition, and sexuality. We are keenly aware that our values and beliefs have been shaped by these positions. Striving to continuously develop the practice of allyship with historically oppressed and marginalized identity groups, we work deliberately at understanding how ableism, White-supremacy, heterosexuality, sexism, and classism manifest as institutional practices that marginalize and subordinate others. In this work, we position ourselves as allies, teachers, and scholars whose work is shaped by intersectionality and neurodiversity paradigms.

Social Model of Disability. As Disability Studies in Education scholars, we write this chapter with a social model of disability framework that aims to distinguish between the impairment (biological and functional limitation) and the disability (the social oppression and ableism that results from the category; see Gabel and Connor 2009; Oliver 1990; Shakespeare and Watson 2001). Although the social model of disability is widely recognized in the International Disability Rights Movement, it has had minimal influence over U.S. institutions (including educational, political, or labor) and culture, which view disability through a medical model focused on individual pathology and interventions that attempt to normalize the individual.

Neurodiversity. Neurodiversity as a framework was developed by autistic scholars, community organizers, and activists (Kapp et al. 2013; Walker 2013). Neurodivergent individuals include people who are given labels that indicate their neurology differs from the broader population, such as attention deficit hyperactivity disorder (ADHD), anxiety, depression, or a learning disability (LD), to name a few and values this natural diversity in individual neurology. Our use of a neurodiversity framework calls attention to the perspectives of autistic people and honors their wants and needs. We use this framework as a means of combating ableist notions about autistic people and their sexuality and acknowledge the multiple ways to define healthy sexuality and relationships. Thus, it is understood that autistic development is not pathologized, perceived as a deficit, or in comparison to non-autistic people.

4.4 Chapter Organization

We divided this chapter into sections starting with an overview exploring the research on this topic. Then, risks are discussed as highlighting societal biases and barriers. We move into supports incorporating allies who are not autistic. The topics covered include sexuality and intimacy (including consent, masturbation, and self-advocacy), relationships (flirting, dating, stalking, and abuse), gender and sexuality identity (LGBTQ+ identity, gender identity), sexuality education, and concludes with implications for transition (marriage, partnership, reproduction, raising children, and family). Please note that individuals mentioned here have been de-identified to protect privacy (unless such information is in the public domain).

4.5 Sexuality and Intimacy

4.5.1 Overview

Sexuality is a multi-dimensional individual phenomenon composed of one's sexual, romantic, and intimate thoughts, feelings, and behaviors that shifts and changes over time. Understanding of sexuality develops during puberty, but awareness of attraction, physical differences, and romantic relationships usually occurs in childhood. Autistic individuals face increased barriers to understanding their own sexuality and engaging in intimacy with others due to the complex social expectations that are involved with sexuality. For example, when discussing sexuality, several concepts need to be established prior to considering the technical mechanics of sex, such as sense of self (including autistic identity), body parts, public versus private, various roles and relationships, and respect for others (Reynolds 2013) in order to support a healthy sexual development.

As with other dimensions of sexuality and intimacy, many behaviors and expectations are not often discussed easily, because the taboo nature makes conversations challenging. Parents, teachers, and other allies might be unsure of how to approach such content with young adults. It is important to guide autistic young adults to gain an understanding of sex and sexuality through explicit instruction, clear language, and concrete examples. This is especially true for content considered taboo or part of the "ignored curriculum" (Gougeon 2009), such as masturbation, flirting, etc.

Sexual relationships. For some autistic individuals, sexuality and engaging in sexual behaviors supports connection with other people in meaningful ways that other forms of communication lack. Alternatively, sexual activity can cause significant stress, discomfort, and confusion. For instance, common sensory experiences associated with participating in interpersonal sexual activities can be overwhelming or confusing. Young adults who experience sensory sensitivity would benefit from learning how to advocate for their needs and to set up the terms of such encounters (Groner 2012). As one individual describes:

> I am sensitive to smells and I just can't have sex in a bed that is not clean, but also if the sheets have been washed in a strong smelling washing powder or liquid. In both cases, I just get fixated on the smell and lose all interest in sex as I just want to get out of there. I found the best way to manage this and still have any kind of sex life is to only have sex in my house in my bed. I wash the sheets myself so I know they are clean and smell pleasant, which means I am not preoccupied with smelling sheets and so can focus on touch and feel and move more easily into sex. -Tony (Goodall 2016).

4.5.2 Risks and Barriers

Without explicitly addressing norms, values, and experiences around sexuality, young autistic adults face higher risk of behaviors that mark them as deviant (public disrobing, sexual unrequited obsession with other people, public masturbation, etc.), put them or others in unsafe situations (unwanted pregnancies, sexual abuse, aggression, involvement in the judicial system as sex offenders, etc.), or act as a barrier to achieving a meaningful romantic and sexual life.

Consent. Giving and receiving consent is a vital concept to speak about with all young adults to prepare for navigating healthy sexual or intimate encounters. For autistic young adults, conversations about consent involve detailed conversations around boundaries, which can be explicitly taught. Dr. Kofke once worked with a 16-year-old autistic adolescent, Leo, who had an affinity for specific clothing that related to his sexual preferences. At school he would reach out and lightly touch the clothing of familiar female students. A few young women tolerated this behavior; however, Leo's family became increasingly concerned about the issue of consent. Dr. Kofke and Leo's family framed boundaries as a personal bubble, engaged in perspective taking of what it would feel like to have clothing touched without asking, discussed circumstances when it would be appropriate to touch clothing (after being in an established relationship with the person and talking about it first), and alternative means of engaging in this sexual preference, like looking at photos of the clothing online. Revisiting these lessons with Leo weekly was a necessary component to the application of consent.

Illegal sexual behaviors. Although autistic individuals are more likely than their neurotypical peers to be victims of sexual misconduct, there is a rising focus on legal problems linked to sexual behavior (Attwood et al. 2014; see also Dubin, Chap. 9). These issues include sexual acts performed publicly, illegal consumption of pornography, and involvement with sex-workers. Where and when masturbation can occur, what kind of pornography is safe to consume (and where), the meaning of paying for sexual behavior with others, and how engaging in online sexual activity does not equate with real life interests, are taboo topics that *must* be discussed explicitly. Without this guidance, autistic individuals could lose their jobs, be isolated from social experiences, and (at worst case) be incarcerated.

Dr. Kahn once consulted with a teacher whose autistic student, Aiden, exchanged video games and money for friendship when he was younger. He was never explicitly taught otherwise. As Aiden grew older (he was over 18), he exchanged money and valuables for sexual favors from his neurotypical under aged classmates. Due to the legal severity of the situation, he was arrested and charged with very serious crimes. This could have been avoided if Aiden was given appropriate knowledge and skills for dating and sexuality. In another case (as explored by Dubin, Chap. 9), a young man with Aspergers, Nick Dubin, received the recommendation by his therapist to explore his sexuality through viewing pornographic materials. Nick was arrested for downloading (and distributing) child pornography without the knowledge of what he did wrong. Nick's arrest and eventual conviction could have been avoided if he had been explicitly instructed on safe and moral outlets for consuming erotic material (Attwood et al. 2014).

4.5.3 Supports

In addition to meaningful sexual education, there are other important dimensions for supporting the sexual development of a young autistic adult. First, critically examine what beliefs, values, and foundational knowledge the young adult has already developed. Also, know what your own limitations are regarding knowledge and values so that you can find specific resources to support the individual in a way that honors their unique desires, strengths, and needs. Other ways to support autistic individuals include sharing knowledge about self-stimulation, and promoting self-advocacy and self-agency.

Masturbation and pornography. Masturbation (or self-stimulation) is a common sexual activity that is rarely discussed with teachers, caregivers, and family members due to the taboo nature of the subject or "the societal belief that it is either shameful or private" (Hingsburger 1994). As many autistic individuals are visual learners who benefit from explicit explanations, this failure to discuss taboo topics can manifest in difficult outcomes that are associated with sexual frustration. These outcomes could occur from a lack of understanding of public and private, lack of sexual opportunities, pleasure derived from self-stimulation, or even from a developed routine (e.g. undressing or using a restroom). Some helpful direct examples can be useful, such as social stories with explicit language ("touching your vulva" vs. "masturbation") or appropriate visual representation (such as a "how-to" film; Hingsburger 1994). Also, the avoidance of unrealistic images (such as commercial pornography) can be helpful as those images can be confusing and problematic.

Autistic young adults succeed best in an environment with predictability and explicitness. Allies can provide the needed structure and accommodations to support the young adult. Masturbation fulfills various functions for all individuals, including pleasure, gratification, relaxation, assistance with sleep, entertainment, and relief from anxiety, depression, or even anger (Reynolds 2013). It is only considered inappropriate when it occurs in public (or in private without the consent of others present), causes self-injury, and when frequency interferes with daily living (Hingsburger 1994).

Dr. Kahn once worked with Marco, a 20-year-old non-speaking autistic young man with an intellectual disability. One morning the school office called to let her know Marco was being sent home after exposing himself and masturbating on the school bus. This was not the first time this had happened, nor was it the only location. Marco was receiving extended special education services in a self-contained classroom focused on transition skills with community interaction and work experience education. Dr. Kahn realized that all of the transition skills and supports they were working on would be for naught if this behavior continued. Working with his parents, albeit initially uncomfortable as they identified as from a very modest culture, they provided educational supports through visual cues and explicit routines such as door hangers requesting privacy in the bathroom and bedroom, a timer for a set duration, and a post-masturbation hygiene routine, so Marco would have an outlet for his desires and feelings as well as education around appropriate and safe behaviors. With this system in place, the inappropriate behavior ceased while supporting Marco's needs.

Pornography consumption can also provide individuals with sexual engagement when used appropriately and safely. Research has shown, however, that people who consume increased levels of pornography develop the belief that individuals engage in everyday sexual behaviors reflected in pornography (Beddows and Brooks 2016). It is important for autistic individuals to understand that, even though this might be one of the only visual representations of sexual behaviors that they have seen, the sexual behaviors shown in pornographic representations are not how most people engage in sexual relationships (Goodall 2016).

4.6 Relationships

4.6.1 Overview

Historically, a pervasive stereotype about autistic people suggests a lack of empathy and preference for social isolation. Recent research and writing by autistic people show much evidence to the contrary: autistic people want to engage deeply with others and have close relationships (Jaswal and Akhtar 2019). Often, the issue resides in neurotypical people's misunderstandings about autistic behavior, and vice versa (Rosqvist 2014). This can lead to increased isolation and loneliness for autistic people, which may result in mental health issues. Recent evidence suggests that autistic people create stronger bonds of understanding with other autistic people and feel minoritized when in relationships with non-autistic people (Crompton et al. 2019).

Research recommends that fostering peer relationships leads to increased knowledge about friendship and romantic relationships (Hancock et al. 2017). Discussion about relationships, dating, and sexual activity occurs informally in friendship circles.

Inclusion in this ignored curriculum is important as autistic youth are more susceptible to being bullied by their peers and often miss out on these kinds of conversations. Sparrow R. Jones (2017) describes how the bullying she underwent from her peers created a misunderstanding of appropriate sexual activity:

> When I was in middle school, the bullying I had been subject to for the last six or seven years suddenly took on a sexual tone. The girls bullied me by spreading rumors that I was having sex, by calling me sexual names, including ones I didn't even understand yet, by drawing obscene pictures of me or writing obscene notes about me and passing the around the room so they would make their way to me, then giggling when I saw them.
>
> The boys bullied me too, but in a different way. I got pulled into niches beneath the stairs or little alcoves behind the lockers where I would be groped or kissed against my will-disgusting, wet kisses with tongue. (p. 81)

Jones' experience highlights how relationships with peers may create misunderstandings about healthy sexual behavior that supports a burgeoning sexuality. When autistic students are absent from appropriate friendship conversations, they miss out on learning crucial information about permissible sexual behavior for themselves and their romantic partners.

4.6.2 Risks and Barriers

Autistic young adults are vulnerable to relational victimization and can be unintentional sexual offenders. As people with developmental disabilities, they are at an increased risk of sexual victimization in both childhood (Edelson 2010) and adulthood (Brown-Lavoie et al. 2014). Conversely, autistic adolescents are at an increased risk of engaging in less appropriate sexual behavior, and less likely to adhere to sexual privacy norms (Hancock et al. 2017).

Sedgewick et al. (2019) studied the relational experiences of autistic women and compared those experiences to non-autistic counterparts. There was a higher rate of sexual abuse and victimization reported by the autistic women. This occurred because the autistic women in the study were more likely to continue to engage with potential sexual partners, who misread flirtatious cues as an invitation for a sexual encounter, which may not always be the intent. Although it should not be the responsibility of any woman advocate for her consent, without understanding how to convey her consent to sexual activity, autistic women in the study experienced more abusive situations when dating. Flirting, stalking and sexual victimization are briefly discussed here as notable risks related to the vulnerability of autistic young adults.

Flirting. Television, the Internet, and pornography may be consulted in order to learn about dating rituals, such as flirting and gaining the attention of a romantic interest (Brown-Lavoie et al. 2014). Such sources are not always accurate portrayals of the expected interaction. In the study by Sedgewick and colleagues (2019), autistic women reported they tended to learn about dating behavior through fantastical portrayals in media outlets. These observations lead to highly sexualized flirting attempts while dating. The other person misunderstood the intent behind a highly flirtatious act and attempted to engage in sexual activity, which resulted in a freeze response from the autistic woman and eventual sexual abuse.

Stalking. Autistic individuals may pursue their romantic interest for a long period of time. Their interests could involve much interaction with the individual, or sometimes they will attempt to pursue a person they have admired from afar. This phenomenon occurs when autistic people are engaged in few relationships with others, misunderstand how stalking behavior is perceived by others or how to otherwise engage in appropriate courtship rituals (Stokes et al. 2007).

Sexual victimization. In a survey completed by Brown-Lavoie et al. (2014) compared to non-autistic peers, autistic people are 3 times more likely to experience unwanted sexual contact, 2.7 times more likely to experience sexual coercion, and 2.4 times more likely to experience forced intercourse. Both men and women experienced forms of sexual victimization. The decreased level of sexual knowledge in autistic individuals may account for this increased rate of sexual victimization, as do perceived language and social-emotional barriers that can lead autistic young adults to become more targeted victims (Edelson 2010).

4.6.3 Supports

Relational supports and sexual well-being for autistic youth largely reside in effective social and communication skills (Byers et al. 2013). Starting in adolescence, autistic youth need access to friendships to talk about sexual activity. The general population also needs to be informed about misunderstandings that can occur when engaging in relationships with autistic people. Specifically, how autistic people's behavior when flirting or pursuing a romantic interest may not always align with neurotypical norms for such behavior.

Post et al. (2014) provide strategies for educating autistic students about stalking behavior, which includes discussion of self-regulation strategies through social stories and video modeling. Awareness of the high rates of sexual abuse for autistic women also needs to be openly discussed as well as how to safely approach dating and examples of consent to sexual activity. Victims should know that *any* instance of sexual abuse *is not their fault*. Searching the hashtag #MeToo to learn about the stories of sexual assault victims may assist with proactive support as well as understanding the psychological effects that occur after an abusive sexual interaction. If sexual abuse has occurred, seeking psychological assistance with a professional who has experience working with autistic individuals who have undergone trauma is preferable.

The research community needs to keep track of sexual victimization of autistic people and maintain up-to-date reports (Brown-Lavoie et al. 2014). There is a lack of current reporting on sexual victimization of autistic people, who may be lumped into the larger category of sexual victimization of people with developmental disabilities (ASAN 2015). In this area, the largest support would be for legal researchers to include specific disability labels and to continue to publish case studies on the sexual victimization of this population.

4.7 Gender and Sexual Identity

4.7.1 Overview

Autistic young adults experience gender and sexuality in a more fluid manner than neurotypical counterparts. Davidson and Tamas (2016) clarify this concept from the perspectives of autistic people:

> Since our earliest conversations on the subject [of gender], we've been aware of and increasingly bothered by the sense of gender as a ghostly presence/ absence ... something that autistic accounts reveal to be there, but not really; something that slips in and out of their awareness, that's felt to circulate around but never quite settle in their lives, or on their bodies, and never shapes their interactions in quite the way it's supposed to. (p. 61)

We understand gender and sexuality as residing beyond traditional binary measures (e.g. male/female, heterosexual/homosexual). One's gender may not align with his/her/their biological sex. Also, the sexuality and gender of individuals is subject to change depending on their personal identity and personal preferences for describing their gender and sexuality. Keeping this sociocultural construction of gender and sexuality in mind is imperative to understanding how autistic people perceive these components of their identities. We approach the use of binary gender terms, like female/male with the understanding that a person's gender identity can be separate from the genitalia they were born with, as well as identifying beyond the gender binary as a person with non-binary or agender identities.

There is also a very high overlap of identification as transgender and autism (George and Stokes 2018). In fact, Kahn and Lindstrom (2015) found that male autistic young adults often did not feel the same constraints concerning gender norms, feeling freer to act in ways that suited them, and not be confined to societal expectations of being male. Autistic females have a higher likelihood of identifying across the gender binary and lower rates of heterosexual preference (May et al. 2017). Often, autistic people have a more nuanced understanding of gender with a higher number of autistic individuals identifying beyond male or female as gender- neutral, agender, non-binary, or have a non-traditional sense of gender identity (Jack 2014). There may be frustration at the lack of ability to express their sense of gender, or feel that the social gender roles are viewed as too rigid and need to be more flexible. Sexual preference is also understood to be beyond straight or homosexual to pansexual, bisexual, asexual, and/or polyamorous.

The disproportionate gender discrepancy in autism diagnosis is another issue related to gender. More males are diagnosed with autism than females. Current prevalence of rates of autism, as determined by the Centers for Disease Control and Prevention (2019) determine 1:39 males at the age of 8 are diagnosed with autism, compared with 1:151 females. One issue arising from this gender-based diagnosis is the phenomenon of autistic girls and women discovering their diagnosis much later than their male counterparts. It is common for autistic women to discover that they are autistic well into adulthood, and only after first being given a veritable menu of other mental disorder diagnoses (e.g. anxiety, anorexia, obsessive compulsive disorder, depression, bi-polar disorder, attention-deficit hyperactivity disorder, learning disability, etc.).

4.7.2 Risks and Barriers

It is common for autistic people to have co-existing mental health issues, which can have much impact on their daily life. One of the most common issues is anxiety and depression due to attempts to be as neurotypical as possible, which is also known as masking or camouflaging autism. While this also occurs in autistic boys and men, it is common for autistic girls and women to start masking from a very early age, which can delay receiving appropriate services or diagnoses. Autistic women often learn dating rituals and learning how to perform femininity from watching media outlets. As described in the relationships section, this kind of masking can lead to sexual victimization and misunderstandings about how to state consent.

With regard to the high rates of transgender identity and autism, there is an increased likelihood of relational and sexual victimization in the transgender population.

Barriers include the feminization of identification as a victim, as well as access to appropriate resources when transgender people are the victims of intimate partner relationships (Guadalupe-Diaz and Jasinski 2017). This can be a substantial barrier for transgender people who are not autistic, as most resources are gender-specific and do not seem to understand the unique needs of the transgender population. Navigating these social support systems without assistance may be very difficult for transgender autistic individuals.

4.7.3 Supports

Emerging research focuses on the crucial need for autistic mentorship relationships to better understand the nuances involved with gender and autism. Ninja, age 15, stated the following about her understanding of autism (Kofke 2019):

> Well. I've heard that autistic women, like myself, tend to be kind of shy. You know. Or they might be a bit irritable…Kind of like me…considering the fact that I don't really understand, like the difference between autistic women and autistic men quite yet. Like I guess ah. Not sure. I just, I just know. I'm not an expert, you know. (p. 135)

Ninja had been exposed to resource books about autism and had not yet read a memoir or blog written by an autistic person, let alone another autistic woman. Without support from autistic mentors, she felt like she did not know enough about autism and wondered about an intersection with autism and gender. Autistic mentors (either in person or online) can allow autistic young adults authentic role model relationships to have supportive conversations about sexuality and gender.

Providing autistic youth and young adults with autistic narratives can be another avenue for gender and sexuality support (Jones 2017). Temple Grandin's identity as asexual, John Elder Robinson's lessons from his marriages, or Dawn Prince-Hughe's self-realization of her lesbian identity are examples of autistic stories that promote a range of different perspectives on sexuality and relationships. Searching for autistic blogs discussing gender identity and experiences with sexual and relational victimization. The Genderbread Person (see Appendix) is an online tool developed for personal and educational use, which explicitly discusses understanding the intersections of gender identity, gender expression, and biological sex as a continuum and can be very helpful when explicitly teaching various dimensions of our identity.

4.8 Sexuality Education

4.8.1 Overview

Due to the taboo nature of sexuality, assumptions prevail that an autistic child does not want/need information about sexuality, or teaching a child about sex will increase their sexual activity. On the contrary, Kirby (2007), with the National Campaign to Prevent Teen Pregnancy, found that greater parent–child communication about sex and contraception is a strong protective factor for lower rates of teen pregnancy and sexually transmitted infection (STI) transmission. For autistic individuals, it is especially important that communication accommodates their individual needs.

Sexuality education (sex ed) occurs across formal and informal settings. It is often offered in U.S. public schools as part of state-mandated health and wellness curriculum. Despite the opportunity for sex ed in school, autistic youth are still at risk for increased sexual misconduct or victimization. Since neurotypical peers tend to learn about sex and sexuality through the ignored curriculum, autistic youth are at a disadvantage without this informal peer education. In the absence of established closely connected friendship networks, families tend to take on a larger sex ed role. This potentially places parents in an uncomfortable position of having frank discussions about sex and sexuality when talking with autistic youth and young adults.

4.8.2 Risks and Barriers

Although sex ed is formally introduced in the public-school system, students who are in segregated special education classrooms in their public schools have a decreased likelihood of attending such classes. Even if autistic students can participate in formal sex education, sex may be discussed from an ableist perspective assuming disabled people are not sexual beings. Special educators need access to professional development in order to effectively teach sex ed in schools (Curtiss and Ebata 2016). Autistic students might not identify or agree with sex ed curricula that frames gender and sexuality as binaries (female/male, homosexual/heterosexual (Davidson and Tamas 2016; Jack 2014).

When families are responsible for educating their autistic youth and young adults about sex and sexuality, they find it challenging to make their conversations relevant to the autistic individual. Families may also insert their bias regarding sex and disability into the conversation, and limit the possibilities for their autistic person (Holmes et al. 2016). This limited education can lead to misunderstandings about sex and sexuality. Families that are uncomfortable with these conversations may abandon them altogether. An unfortunate result of this discomfort is autistic youths' increased engagement in at-risk sexual behavior and learning about dating and sex from unrealistic depictions found in media sources.

4.8.3 Supports

Starting in preadolescence, autistic youth need explicit education about sex and sexuality. When families are primarily responsible for this education, they need to consider using autistic-friendly methods in addition to talking. Such methods include the use of visual aids, books, and social stories (Holmes et al. 2016). When families educate their autistic youth about sex, they often focus on sexual hygiene and privacy. While important, families also need to include topics on sexuality, gender, and relationships (Hartmann et al. 2019). This can occur in school or through family-based services. When families engage in family-based sex ed curricula, they report a higher comfort level with the content and with talking about it with their autistic person.

Any sex education needs to incorporate concepts related to sexuality and gender as well as understanding the difference between abusive behavior and flirting. Undoubtedly all students, autistic or neurotypical, will benefit from such discussion. Additionally, the best way for autistic people to learn about issues surrounding sex is through their close social contacts. The best support for autistic people lies in fostering authentic friendships where they can comfortably discuss sex and sexuality. Education in settings dedicated to inclusive supports can increase access to peer socialization about dating and romance (Brown-Lavoie et al. 2014).

Additional education is needed in areas like sexuality and consent (Barnett and Maticka-Tyndale 2015), the behaviors that are considered sexually abusive, either as a victim or an abuser, and the consequences to such behavior. The online resource Sex Education for Self-Advocates! published by the Organization for Autism Research (see Appendix) is designed to help autistic young adults become self-advocates and learn about the multiple dimensions of sexuality and relationships including consensual sexual encounters, online dating, and knowing when you are ready to engage in sexual activities. The Birds and the Bees curriculum (see Appendix) is an example of a free curriculum resource developed to support the sexual education of autistic youth and young adults.

In addition, for students who received specially designed instruction under their Individualized Education Plan (IEP), issues of sexuality, gender, sexual orientation, etc. could be incorporated into their IEP. Appropriate sex education could be included as a transition goal for students 14 and over (Frith et al. 1981) in order to establish sex education as a need for successful transition. For students who have barriers to social relationships and social environments, but who still might want to participate in a Gay Straight Alliance or other similar student club, an IEP can support their ability to participate (Kahn and Lindstrom 2015). As sexuality and identity development is so closely linked to meaningful transitions to adulthood, transition goals on an IEP would be a great place to provide these supports.

4.9 Implications for Transition to Adulthood

This chapter was written to explain the dimensions of sexuality and how to assist autistic young adults while supporting their unique needs and strengths as they transition to adulthood. As with the other dimensions of the transition to adult life described in this book, desires, preferences, and needs should be completely based upon the individual's preferences. This is crucial for achieving a high quality of life, feeling safe and secure in one's home and community, and maintaining a sense of meaning for the individual. Quality of life can often connect to outcomes such as marriage, partnership, and parenthood. The research on marriage and parenting for autistic people is limited. The research that does exist is often founded in deficit paradigms of disability, causing further damage to the autistic community by supporting biases, discrimination, and ableist treatment while ignoring their autonomy.

***Marriage, partnership,* etc.** All relationships, regardless of disability, require work around communication and expectations. For many autistic individuals, barriers in communication and understanding the social cues of their partners can lead to challenges in committed relationships. All individuals in a relationship, whether they identify as autistic or not, should be committed to developing a communication system that works for both parties in order to express their emotions, beliefs, and desires in the relationship, whether they are married or not.

Although there are several financial benefits to marriage (tax breaks, etc.) it is important to be aware of funding disincentives as well. Being married to someone who works can change qualifications and benefits for various programs (see Doyle, Chap. 1). For example, if one depends on Supplemental Security Income (SSI) the addition of a spouse's income and assets most likely disqualifies someone from receiving the income-dependent benefit. This gets complicated if two people who both receive SSI marry each other. This can also be true for their Medicaid benefits. However, for those receiving benefits from Social Security Disability Insurance (SSDI), they can often keep their full benefits as they are not means-based (if the benefits are under their own working record). Social Security's policies around marriage are complex and vary by state. If you have questions, the best sources would be the local Social Security Administration office or a legal professional. Although people with disabilities have the right to marry, these financial considerations can significantly influence a person's decision to do so.

Reproduction, raising children, and family. Although we know that autistic parents are not significantly different from neurotypical parents, discrimination against parents with disabilities is common throughout society as well as the legal system. Stereotyping of autistic parents as lacking empathy or uncaring, despite research discrediting these claims, have persisted in guiding family law professionals. Consequently, some autistic people claim that, "fear of discrimination in child custody proceedings keeps them from leaving relationships with abusive partners" (National Council on Disabilities 2012). The child welfare system is not prepared to support parents with disabilities and their families, contributing to increasingly high rates of involvement with child welfare services. Within the system, parents with disabilities regularly encounter discriminatory practices. This issue affects many parents with disabilities in adulthood, so much so that the United Nations Convention on the Rights of Persons with Disabilities (which the United States has not ratified), stresses the rights of people with disabilities to create and maintain families without ableist discrimination (UN General Assembly 2007).

Family planning looks different for all prospective parents; however, autistic individuals seeking fertility treatment or adoption face additional barriers. There is a long history of ill treatment and ableism in the area of procreation and parenting for individuals with disabilities (including a long history of forced sterilization) (National Council on Disability 2012). Because of unclear policies regarding fertility treatment and adoption, one's disability could lead to being discriminated against, although it would be difficult to prove and rectify (Mutcherson 2009). The Americans with Disabilities Act does not mandate medical care as a right, but only requires that people with disabilities can seek the same care as a person without disabilities. As for adoption, each agency has criteria that prospective parents must meet, as well as the differing standards mandated by the state, leaving room for differing rules and regulations. For example, in 2011, Virginia approved regulations that allowed agencies to use disability as the sole reason to deny potential parents (National Council on Disability 2012).

Appropriate and explicit instruction on sexual intercourse and contraceptive use supports young adults' autonomy with choices regarding reproduction, pregnancy, and family planning. Autistic people often face additional barriers such as finding a health care provider who is able to effectively support someone with autism, understanding the unpredictable physical changes and sensory experiences of pregnancy and childbirth, or communication barriers. An ally or a self-advocate can assist by searching for resources about reproduction and finding neurodiversity-friendly care providers. After deciding to have a child, autistic people can benefit from classes to prepare them for physical changes, childbirth, sensory experiences, and handling changes in their plans. Seeking out a doula (or birth advocate) who has a background in supporting neurodivergent clients is another option. Alford (2017) encourages doulas to provide online or text resources for communication for clients who find that more accessible, replacing verbal communication during birth when "typically the social/language part of the brain becomes harder to access as labor intensifies," and a plan for sensory overload that will be addressed in the individual's birth plan.

Many autistic parents view their unique strengths as an important dimension to their parenting:

> My wife and I wanted children because we wanted to give a child a better life than we had as aspies growing up when the world did not understand...it was very overwhelming when we had three kids under five. But both of us love exploring the world with our kids, getting excited by looking for bugs in the garden or learning how to cook pancakes. -Dean (Goodall 2016)

As with all parents, it is important to identify the parents' strengths and needs for support so that they can be connected with appropriate resources and support networks. Lightfoot & DeZelar (2020) introduce parent-centered planning (built on the person-centered planning model) for parents with intellectual and developmental disabilities by building the needed support network and including the parents' desires and goals as parents. To comprehensively understand barriers and supports there needs to be more research completed with the neurodivergent parent community. In addition, it is important for allies to truly listen to the experiences, needs, and joys of autistic people. As O'Toole and Doe (2002) describe:

> In general, with rare exceptions, people with disabilities do not get asked if they want to have children. They don't get asked if they want to be sexual. The silence around sexuality includes their parents, their counselors, their teachers and most health professionals. Yet these same people sometimes counsel in favor of involuntary sterilization.

If we want to effectively support autistic youth as they transition to adulthood, it is vital that we support them along all dimensions of their identities, desires, and personal goals.

4.10 Conclusion

This chapter summarized the most salient aspects related to sexuality and autistic young adults during the transition to adulthood by reviewing sexuality and intimacy, relationships, gender and sexuality identity, sexuality education, and implications for transition. Each section included positive strategies for supporting autistic young adults in their journey to a meaningful and satisfying adult life. We were limited in our lack of discussion about issues of race, religion, culture, language, etc. and the intersectional autistic experience. Autistic people with marginalized and minoritized racial and/or ethnic identities may have very different experiences from those portrayed in this chapter, as diversity of the experiences of autistic people is broad and deep. An appendix of resources aligning with this chapter's focus and promoting a neurodiversity perspective is available in the final pages of this chapter for autistic people, families, educators, and school personnel who want to continue to pursue this topic for their own uses.

As Finger (1992) discussed at the opening of this chapter, it is easier for us to effectively plan for other dimensions of transition for autistic young adults—education, employment, independent living—than it is for us to plan for the part of the transition that is so deeply personal, like sexuality and relationships. We founded this chapter on the importance of supporting and empowering autistic young adults to make healthy and safe decisions that align with their unique strengths and needs and have meaningful transitions to adulthood around sexuality and relationships. As with any other person, autistic people have autonomy and choice in their relationships, as well as unique gender and sexual identities. In presenting this critical perspective, we want readers to consider how to navigate systemic barriers that are rife with ableist assumptions about autism. With much sincerity, we also hope readers of this chapter will follow the wisdom provided by autistic people excerpted here—and the autistic people in their own lives—to truly listen for how to best support sexuality and relationships throughout the transition into adulthood.

Appendix

Resources about sex and sexuality for/by autistic adults

Amaze

https://www.youtube.com/channel/UCXQZTtGgsy6QHH2fg-OJ_eA/featured.

A YouTube channel providing free videos covering a wide range of content related to sex, sexuality and relationships. While not specifically developed for autistic youth, the videos provide a visual support with discussion. The topics are broad, including content like female masturbation, how to communicate effectively, and healthy versus unhealthy relationships. There are also videos developed specifically for families.

The Birds and The Bees

https://asdsexed.org.

Free, online, autistic sex ed curriculum resources for autistic youth and young adults, families and educators. Hot topics include masturbation, sexual health, and sexual safety.

The Genderbread Person

https://www.genderbread.org.

A free, online resource detailing gender, sexuality, and expression using accessible language and colorful visual illustrations to describe these complex and abstract concepts.

The autism spectrum guide to sexuality and relationships: Understand yourself and make choices that are right for you

A guide book that explicitly outlines various dimensions of sexuality and relationships in clear language for Autistic Adults. It is direct and inclusive, using tangible examples, allowing readers to gain expert advice to understand everything from identity, to flirting, finding, maintaining, and ending relationships.

Goodall (2016). *The autism spectrum guide to sexuality and relationships: Understand yourself and make choices that are right for you.* London: Jessica Kingsley.

Scarleteen

https://www.scarleteen.com/article/disability.

Free online resource for teens and young adults to learn all there is to know about sex, sexuality, and relationships. The site demonstrates inclusivity of a broad range of perspectives and has a section dedicated to disability.

Organization for Autism Research's **Sex Ed. for Self-Advocates!** is a sexuality and sex education resource written specifically for people on the autism spectrum age 15 and up. People on the autism spectrum sometimes don't have the chance to learn about sexuality and sex in ways that work for them, so OAR created this guide as a starting point to change that.

https://researchautism.org/sex-ed-guide/.

Zosia Zaks wrote a how to guide from the lens of an autistic woman in order to support a diverse autistic community by providing them tools and explicit explanation of barriers. She also wants to make autistic people more visible in society, increase neurodiversity, and combat ableism. She directly explores issues like, how to cope with sensory challenges on a date, staying safe on internet dating sites,

Zaks, Z. (2006). *Life and love: Positive strategies for autistic adults.* AAPC Publishing.

References

Alford, B. 2017. Respecting neurodiversity in birthwork and language. Doula Training International. https://doulatrainingsinternational.com/respecting-neurodiversity-in-birth-work-and-language/. Accessed 16 Mar 2021

Attwood, T., I. Henault, and N. Dubin. 2014. *The autism spectrum, sexuality and the law: What every parent and professional needs to know*. London: Jessica Kingsley.

Autistic Self-Advocacy Network. 2015. Real Talk Provider Toolkit. https://autisticadvocacy.org/wp-content/uploads/2015/12/Real-Talk-Improving-Quality-of-Sexual-Health-Care-for-Patients-with-Disabilities.pdf. Accessed 16 Mar 2021

Barnett, J.P., and E. Maticka-Tyndale. 2015. Qualitative exploration of sexual experiences among adults on the autism spectrum: Implications for sex education. *Perspectives on Sexual and Reproductive Health 47* (4): 171–179.

Beddows, N., and R. Brooks. 2016. Inappropriate sexual behavior in adolescents with autism spectrum disorder: What education is recommended and why. *Early Intervention in Psychiatry* 10 (4): 282–289.

Brown, L. X. Z. 2012. Autistic Hoya. https://www.autistichoya.com/2012/09/so-high-functioning-sarcasm.html. Accessed 16 Mar 2021

Brown-Lavoie, S.M., M.A. Viecili, and J.A. Weiss. 2014. Sexual knowledge and victimization in adults with autism spectrum disorders. *Journal of Autism and Developmental Disorders* 44 (9): 2185–2196.

Byers, E.S., S. Nichols, S.D. Voyer, and G. Reilly. 2013. Sexual well-being of a community sample of high-functioning adults on the autism spectrum who have been in a romantic relationship. *Autism* 17 (4): 418–433.

Centers or Disease Control and Prevention. 2019. Autism data visualization tool. https://www.cdc.gov/ncbddd/autism/data/index.html. Accessed 16 Mar 2021

Crompton, C.J., S. Fletcher-Watson, D. Ropar. 2019. Autistic peer to peer information transfer is highly effective. https://doi.org/10.31219/osf.io/j4knx

Curtiss, S.L., and A.T. Ebata. 2016. Building capacity to deliver sex education to individuals with autism. *Sexuality and Disability* 34: 27–47. https://doi.org/10.1007/s11195-016-9429-9.

Davidson, J., and S. Tamas. 2016. Autism and the ghost of gender. *Emotion, Space and Society 19*: 59–65. https://doi.org/10.1016/j.emospa.2015.09.009

Edelson, M.G. 2010. Sexual abuse of children with autism: Factors that increase risk and interfere with recognition of abuse. *Disability Studies Quarterly 30* (1).

Finger, A. 1992. Forbidden fruit. *New Internationalist 233*: 8–10.

Frith, G.H., J. Mitchell, and J.D. Lindsey. 1981. Sex education: The neglected dimension on the secondary level individualized education plans. *The Clearing House* 54 (5): 197–199.

Gabel, S. L., & D. J. Connor. 2009. Theorizing disability: Implications and applications for social justice in education. In *Handbook of social justice in education*, 395–417.

George, R., and M.A. Stokes. 2018. Gender identity and sexual orientation in autism spectrum disorder. *Autism* 22 (8): 970–982.

Goodall, E. 2016. *The autism spectrum guide to sexuality and relationships: Understand yourself and make choices that are right for you*. Jessica Kingsley Publishers.

Gougeon, N. 2009. Sexuality education for students with intellectual disabilities, a critical pedagogical approach: Outing the ignored curriculum. *Sex Education 9* (3).

Groner, R. 2012. Sex as "Spock:" autism, sexuality and autobiographical narrative. In *Sex and disability*, ed. R. McRuer, A. Mollow. Duke University Press.

Guadalupe-Diaz, X.L., and J. Jasinski. 2017. "I Wasn't a Priority, I Wasn't Victim" challenges in help seeking for transgender survivors of intimate partner violence. *Violence against Women* 23 (6): 772–792.

Hancock, G.I., M.A. Stokes, and G.B. Mesibov. 2017. Socio-sexual functioning in autism spectrum disorder: A systematic review and meta-analyses of existing literature. *Autism Research* 10 (11): 1823–1833.

Hartmann, K., et al. 2019. Sexuality in the Autism Spectrum Study (SASS): Reports from young adults and parents. *Journal of Autism and Developmental Disorders* 49: 3638–3655. https://doi.org/10.1007/s10803-019-04077-y.

Hingsburger, D. 1994. Masturbation: A consultation for those who support individuals with developmental disabilities. *Canadian Journal of Human Sexuality* 3 (3): 278–282.

Holmes, L., M. Himle, D. Strassberg. 2016. Parental romantic expectations and parent-child sexuality communication in autism spectrum disorders. *Autism: The International Journal of Research and Practice 20* (6), 687–699

Jack, J. 2014. *Autism and gender from refrigerator mothers to computer geeks*. University of Illinois Press.

Jaswal, V. K., and N. Akhtar. 2019. Being versus appearing socially uninterested: Challenging assumptions about social motivation in autism. *Behavioral and Brain Sciences 42.*

Jones, S. R. 2017. Keep her safe; let her fly free. In *What every autistic girl wishes her parents knew*, ed. E.P. Ballou, K. Thomas, and S. daVanport. Autism Women's Network, DragonBee Press.

Kahn, L.G., and L. Lindstrom. 2015. "I just want to be myself": Adolescents with disabilities who identify as a sexual or gender minority. *The Educational Forum* 79 (4): 362–376.

Kapp, S.K., K. Gillespie-Lynch, L.E. Sherman, and T. Hutman. 2013. Deficit, difference, or both? *Autism and Neurodiversity. Developmental Psychology* 49 (1): 59.

Kirby, D. 2007. Research findings on programs to reduce teen pregnancy and sexually transmitted diseases. National Campaign to Prevent Teen Pregnancy.

Kofke, M. 2019. Taking off The mask: Autistic young women's experiences with social skills in high school (Doctoral dissertation). University of Delaware.

Lightfoot, E., and S. DeZelar. 2020. Parent centered planning: A new model for working with parents with intellectual and developmental disabilities. *Children and Youth Services Review 114.*

May, T., K. Pang, and K.J. Williams. 2017. Gender variance in children and adolescents with autism spectrum disorder from the National Database for Autism Research. *International Journal of Transgenderism* 18 (1): 7–15.

Mehzabin, P., and M.A. Stokes. 2011. Self-assessed sexuality in young adults with high-functioning autism. *Research in Autism Spectrum Disorders* 5: 614–621.

Murphy, N.A., and E.R. Elias. 2006. Sexuality of children and adolescents with developmental disabilities. *Pediatrics* 118 (1): 398–403.

Mutcherson, K.M. 2009. Disabling dreams of parenthood: The fertility industry, anti-discrimination, and parents with disabilities. *Law & Inequality* 27: 311.

National Council on Disability. 2012. Rocking the cradle: Ensuring the rights of parents with disabilities and their children. ERIC Clearinghouse.

Oliver, M. 1990. *Politics of disablement*. Macmillan International Higher Education.

O'Toole, C.J., and T. Doe. 2002. Sexuality and disabled parents with disabled children. *Sexuality and Disability* 20 (1): 89–101.

Post, M., L. Haymes, K. Storey, T. Loughrey, and C. Campbell. 2014. Understanding stalking behaviors by individuals with autism spectrum disorders and recommended prevention strategies for school settings. *Journal of Autism and Developmental Disorders* 44 (11): 2698–2706.

Reynolds, K.E. 2013. *Sexuality and severe autism: A practical guide for parents, caregivers and Health educators*. Jessica Kingsley Publishers.

Rosqvist, H.B. 2014. Becoming an 'autistic couple': Narratives of sexuality and couplehood within the Swedish autistic self-advocacy movement. *Sexuality and Disability* 32 (3): 351–363.

Sedgewick, F., L. Crane, V. Hill, and E. Pellicano. 2019. Friends and lovers: The relationships of autistic and neurotypical women. *Autism in Adulthood* 1 (2): 112–123.

Shakespeare, T., and N. Watson. 2001. The social model of disability: An outdated ideology. *Research in Social Science and Disability* 2 (1): 9–28.

Sinclair, J. 2013. Why I dislike "person first" language. *Autonomy, The Critical Journal of Interdisciplinary Autism Studies 1* (2)

Stokes, M., N. Newton, and A. Kaur. 2007. Stalking, and social and romantic functioning among adolescents and adults with autism spectrum disorder. *Journal of Autism and Developmental Disorders* 37 (10): 1969–1986.

UN General Assembly. 2007. Convention on the rights of persons with disabilities: Resolution/adopted by the General Assembly, 24 January 2007, A/RES/61/106.

Walker, N. 2013. Neurocosmopolitanism: Nick Walker's notes on neurodiversity, autism, and cognitive liberty. https://neurocosmopolitanism.com/neuro-what/. Accessed 16 Mar 2021

World Health Organization. 2006. Sexual and reproductive health. www.who.int/reproductivehealth/topics/sexual_health/sh_definitions/en/. Accessed 16 Mar 2021

Chapter 5
Transition and Education

Lillian Peterson and Angelina Strum

Abstract The educational experience for autistic individuals is one that is unique to the individual and their supporting family. There are many factors that encompass best practices, approaches, and choices in planning an educational experience. However, planning for students who are entering their last few years of schooling before adulthood presents unique challenges. This chapter aims to provide an overview of the key factors and considerations in the late stage of the educational process, better known as the transition period. As the process described in this chapter is that of one program in particular, please note that the information provided may only be applicable to a particular subset of autistic individuals.

5.1 Introduction

The educational experience for autistic individuals is one that is unique to the individual and their supporting family. There are many factors that encompass best practices, approaches, and choices in planning an educational experience. However, planning for students who are entering their last few years of schooling before adulthood presents unique challenges. This chapter aims to provide an overview of the key factors and considerations in the late stage of the educational process, better known as the transition period.

In reading this chapter, there are a few notes that should be considered. First, this chapter is an overview. It is by no means meant to capture all of the factors and considerations for every individual. We recognize that the information provided here is limited to a particular subset of autistic individuals who require the supports and services offered by a therapeutic day school. Each state and community may vary in terms of transition supports, adult service options, and the social climate in which individuals live. Several case studies are included throughout the chapter. The case studies are a collection of experiences from students and families and not meant to

L. Peterson · A. Strum (✉)
Giant Steps, Lisle, IL, USA
e-mail: astrum@mygiantsteps.org

N. Elster and K. Parsi (eds.), *Transitioning to Adulthood with Autism: Ethical, Legal and Social Issues*, The International Library of Bioethics 91,
https://doi.org/10.1007/978-3-030-91487-5_5

represent any one specific individual or family. Names and details are fictionalized. In addition, several of the resources used as references were developed by a team of teachers, therapists, educators, and administrators at Giant Steps, a non-profit therapeutic day school in Illinois. These resources have gone through many revisions and edits as the teams and information used to create them have evolved.

One of the most significant themes throughout this chapter is parent and educator advocacy on behalf of the student. When families and educators are informed about autism characteristics, supports, and resources, and have the time and capacity to commit, such advocacy is advantageous. This advantage can make a critical difference. We fully recognize that having access to this level of support is not always available to every student in every community. Therefore, for the sake of discussion, we are presenting best-case options to be taken and the suggestions provided in this chapter are from a 'what's possible' standpoint. We do not go into a deep discussion about other barriers that may impact students and families going through this process but recognize that there is room for further research and discussion related to additional complicating factors.

Lastly, as this is a chapter about the educational process specifically related to the transition into adulthood and post-secondary life, we do not spend a lot of time on educational considerations for earlier periods of time. Significant research and literature has been developed on early intervention and primary education related to autism services and supports. These are extremely important, and we recommend accessing them in conjunction with this chapter, but for our purposes, do not dedicate additional time to highlight those services or strategies.

5.2 What is Transition Planning?

According to the Merriam-Webster Dictionary, the word *transition* when used as a noun is defined as a movement, development, or evolution from one form, stage, or style to another. As a verb, the Merriam-Webster Dictionary defines *transition* as movement from one thing to the next. For many families of individuals with disabilities, the word *transition* does not have a clear definition nor a set starting or end point. The word or stage of *transition* often generates questions and elements of anxiety, rather than concrete answers, even for families who have already spent years advocating and preparing for their child to transition into adulthood. For families who have not prepared for their child's transition, this stage of life is overwhelming with trying to learn and catch up with all the missing pieces of information.

Kaitlin Smith, former Transition Planning Supervisor at Giant Steps Day School, describes transition planning as "the process of establishing a ***coordinated set of activities*** that ultimately create an individualized and detailed road map to reach attainable and agreed-upon outcomes for students and their family." The participants in this process are all the members of the child's educational team. This team includes the parent or guardian, the student, the general education teacher, special education teacher, an expert to communicate any evaluation results, a translator (if needed), and, if wanted, a parent advocate, friend, caregiver, or case manager. The transition plan accompanies the Individualized Education Program (IEP) process and educational goal development. It takes into consideration where students are today and what the educational team's expectations are for their tomorrows. This method enables key stakeholders to create an individualized life plan for how the student can exit the school system and enter adulthood successfully.

Throughout this process, 3 essential questions should be continuously asked by educators and families as guideposts for navigating the special education and transition roadmap:

1. How will the student's strengths and interests best be accessed in a post-secondary environment?
2. In order for the student to positively and productively engage in their community with the highest level of independence possible, what additional skills or opportunities need to be fostered or created?
3. What resources and support system will be in place for the autistic adult and how will that influence their post-secondary outcomes?

5.3 Timing of Transition Planning

The educational process for individuals with special needs is not a one size fits all process. The road map for each individual student is unique. In order to help students and their families best prepare for this, we recommend starting to think about and outline the needs of transition planning in mid to late elementary school. Below is a simple example outlining the steps related to paperwork, exploring adult program options, and the financial components that should accompany the educational process. Differences may exist from community to community. A more comprehensive list is included in Appendix 1 and more in-depth discussion can be found in the contributing chapters in this book.

When?	What?
Elementary—as early as possible (Summer before Junior High at the latest)	Register for PUNS(Prioritization for Urgency of Need for Services - Illinois) or Medicaid Waiver application program in your state Start reading and learning about SSI (income dependent until 18) Visit at least one adult day program, adapted vocational setting, or supported college facility designed to support autistic adult individuals Complete a special needs trust
Elementary/Junior High	Look into SSI (income dependent until 18) 1 additional visit to an adult day program, adapted vocational setting, or supported college facility designed to support autistic adult individuals Complete a special needs trust

(continued)

(continued)

When?	What?
High School/Transition 4–6 years prior to exit	Obtain State ID Register for publictransportationridership
High school (once 18) and transition 4–5 years prior to exit	Apply for SSI Obtainguardianship, power of attorney, conservatorship, or sign relevant releases of information pending the needed support of the autistic student Schedule transition meeting with the educational team 1 additional visit to an adult day program, adapted vocational setting, or supported college facility designed to support autistic adult individuals
Transition 3 years prior to exit	1 additional visit to an adult day program, adapted vocational setting, or supported college facility designed to support autistic adult individuals Schedule transition meeting with the educational team
Transition 2 years prior to exit	Apply for Medicaid 1 additional visit to an adult day program, adapted vocational setting, or supported college facility designed to support autistic adult individuals Schedule transition meeting with the educational team
Transition 1 year prior to exit	Complete letter of intent 1 additional visit to an adult day program, adapted vocational setting, or supported college facility designed to support autistic adult individuals Schedule transition meeting with the educational team
Transition Exit year	Map out a schedule that outlines the projected timing, resources, and support plan for each day/week of the students anticipated post-secondary schedule @2021 Giant Steps IL

Alongside the process of financial planning and investigating what program options are available, the transition planning process requires the educational team to develop the Transition Plan and education goals that bolster that plan. The U.S. Department of Education's Individuals with Disabilities Education Act (IDEA) (2004) requires that transition planning starts by the time the student reaches age sixteen. Many states recommend or require an even earlier starting age than sixteen. As stated before, laying the foundation for a student's educational, vocational, and intended outcomes should start well before the child reaches their teens. Starting the planning process by considering where a parent sees the student in the future based on identified strengths, abilities, foreseeable limitations, and family goals is helpful. If a parent can conceptualize what the desired outcomes are for their child prior to the age of twenty-two or the indicated school exit date it will make the "backward chaining" method of transition planning much easier and allow for adjustments to the plan along the way. The transition planning process should incorporate a backward timeline of desired outcomes such as ten years from now, 5 years from now, 2 years from now, and 6 months from now for example.

Naomi

Naomi is a kind and playful young autistic adult. She was in a transition program in her late teens. Naomi had limited expressive verbal communication, often answering questions with the same one or two words. She could follow short simple written directions and was able to complete familiar vocational tasks such as sorting, assembling materials, or cleaning, but would often become distracted or disinterested within the first few minutes of the work. When given the choice Naomi would choose to listen to music, play with her favorite stuffed animals, or walk around and check out what her peers were working on throughout class. Naomi was the daughter of two professionally successful parents. Their family values included celebrating hard work, accessing higher education, and gaining financial independence. Their eldest daughters Denise and Malikah had both completed high school and four year college programs with high honors. They each had managed to save enough money through traditional work options post college that they had moved out of their parents' home and moved into a shared apartment together and managed their own bills and schedules. Denise was actively applying for graduate school and Malikah had recently received a promotion at work.

This more traditional path along with such financial and professional stability is an ambitious goal for any young adult and Naomi's parents were very proud of her siblings. Their experience with their older children set a tone for what their hopes and goals were for Naomi's future and made it initially complicated to accept that Naomi's path may not be so straightforward.

The work of the IEP team was to help outline what Naomi's strengths and learning deficits were and how they could help map out realistic goals for her future, while keeping the family goals in mind. Initially Naomi's diagnosis of being on the autism spectrum and having a cognitive impairment were very difficult for the family to accept. Specifically, when Naomi would get upset at home, she would often cry or yell at her family members or an inanimate object. The family, while disliking this response, had the most difficulty accepting that this was a sign of a gap in self-regulation and communication skills and not simply an act of defiance on Naomi's part. Additionally, each annual progress report meeting felt tense and often the family left frustrated and disappointed at the level of progress they felt the educational team was making with Naomi.

To help address this disconnect between the family and the school team, several cross-over meetings were held. These meetings included the parents, social worker, teacher, and administrator. The school team asked the family to describe what their hopes were for Naomi and more about the family dynamic. After learning about the family's values and background, the school team was better able to explain the skills that they were seeing at school with Naomi and how they envisioned those skills expanding over time. They were able to collaborate with the family to identify potential outcomes for her that were vocationally oriented and addressed self-advocacy skills. Using the format of backward chaining was especially helpful for the family, because it was logical, clear, and aligned with their strategic nature.

Once they were able to accept that Naomi's future may not look exactly like her sisters', they were then able to adjust their end goal to one that better suited Naomi. By hearing the parents' concerns and understanding the value system, the educational team could shift from feeling defensive at the annual meetings to arrange for strategies and goal development planning that worked in conjunction with the family. In the end, Naomi's parents' drive pushed the school team to expand their assumptions about her capabilities, and the school team's adjustment in communication helped the parents shift their understanding of Naomi's autism so that they could better support the stepping stones she was making when they didn't always happen in a linear fashion. For Naomi, the focus on the skills below helped to increase her independence and increased her positive relationships both at home, in her community volunteer setting, and at school.

- Increasing Vocational Skills by:
  - Being able to ask for help when needed
  - Being able to increase the amount of time she could attend to a task without needing a break or becoming distracted
  - Increasing the ability to state when she was finished with a given task
- Increasing her Self-Advocacy Skills by:
  - Gaining a person's (e.g. parent, teacher, staff's) attention when she needed something
  - Stating calmly that she did not like something or wanted something to change (e.g. "Could you change the music?").

The outcome of this collaboration was that Naomi attended a therapeutic day school through high school and part of her transition program, and then moved into a program that provided increased vocational opportunities in more diverse community settings (e.g. office tasks, hospitality, and medical centers). This shift was made possible due to her progress and gave both her and the family a sense of pride and accomplishment that matched their family goals and expanded Naomi's options for her post-transition experience.

The transition plan itself is a document within an IEP for students 14 ½ through the day before the child's 22nd birthdate (the maximum eligible age for education services in Illinois). The key elements of the transition plan includes result-oriented future outcomes in 4 key areas:

1. **Employment**: Will the adult obtain competitive employment? Supported employment? Volunteer placement?
2. **Education**: Will the adult attend a four year or community college, participate in a vocational certification program, or need continued development with functional academics/life skills?
3. **Training**: Will the adult need hands-on job training? Development of interview skills? Practice of new skills to apply in an unfamiliar setting?
4. **Independent Living Skills**: Will the adult live independently or in a group setting? Know how to cook and complete daily hygiene routines? Be able to self-regulate or communicate daily needs and wants?

This document is created in conjunction with the annual summary of progress and development of individualized educational goals. It is meant to be an evolving document that gets reviewed, reflected on, and edited regularly. As the student develops and progresses across their educational career and parents and families gain more insight about what options may be available or preferred for their child in the post-twenty-two world, the long-term outcome goals may change. As the long-term picture shifts, so too should the related transition plan and IEP goals.

The idea of long-term planning can be a very difficult concept to tackle when the child is still in elementary school, especially for an autistic student. Often the student and the educational team are still developing foundational skills, practicing expectations for even being in a classroom, and working diligently to establish a working and successful behavior plan for the current placement and environment. If the transition planning process is seen as a marathon and not as a sprint, families and educators can develop partnerships early that focus on building essential skills systematically, strategically, and are meaningfully based on the cognitive and physical developmental stages of the individual. When viewed as a process that can evolve over time and is complementary to the ongoing IEP, it can help to diffuse some of the surrounding anxiety about the timing and intensity of transition planning.

5.4 Linking Educational Goals to the Transition Plan

In developing IEPs and transition plans with goals that best prepare a student for increased independence, the ability for the student to access their community in a functional and meaningful way and the opportunity to have positive interpersonal relationships is key. Knowing that the student may also be in an adapted setting due to the intensity or dynamic nature of their autism, it is also imperative that as the child ages the educational team assess how the accommodations, supports, and adapted environment that have been provided for the child to increase their educational progress will be faded or adjusted to translate into the future outcome goals and placement for the post-school setting.

As the IEP goals are created and the big picture vision evolves, the student's strengths, interests, and own personal goals should be at the forefront of the conversation. Depending on the child, this may take creativity and patience from the teachers, therapists, and family to hone in on what the child wants for themselves, and to determine the strengths that will be most relevant to their future planning. The most efficient way to assess what specific goals should be developed is to identify where the student rates in relation to their most essential skills.

Below is an Essential Skills List developed by various stakeholders within the educational setting that include school administrators, teachers, and therapists led by the not-for-profit Giant Steps. This Essential Skills List is an outline of identified skills that are needed to increase an individual's potential for independence and are applicable to a wide range of students and abilities from kindergarten through adulthood. The purpose of identifying key essential skills as the basis for IEP goal development is to give individuals the tools necessary to reduce maladaptive behavior and foster independence. This list was specifically developed for autistic individuals who are seeking to maximize skills that will increase their success in adult day program settings, supported employment and volunteer opportunities, and who may have challenges adjusting from a highly structured environment into a less predictable and less individualized setting. We recommend using the guide as a tool across the entire educational team, including related service therapists and experts. When it is referenced as part of an inter-disciplinary approach it allows for several benefits to manifest:

- *Accountability*—Ensures that all IEP team members are considering the same foundational skills as having similar value and weight in determining long term success for the student
- *Common Language*—Provides uniformity in the language that the team is using when discussing student needs and progress
- *Holistic Approach*—Helps each service provider think about all relevant areas of student performance, needs, supports, and projected outcomes, not just the ones that apply to their discipline
- *Informed Decision-Making*—Allows for ease of communicating data across teams as a student transitions out of and into new classrooms, due to consistent base measuring tool across the schooling career of the student

Key Essential Skills

1. Possesses and utilizes an identified reliable, spontaneous communication method
2. Demonstrates self-management behavior
3. Safely participates in groups of 5+ individuals
4. Completes personal care routines independently
5. Follows spoken and visual directions
6. Respects and maintains appropriate boundaries of self and others (physical and social)
7. Follows directions from multiple people
8. Manages bodily functions independently
9. Demonstrates choice making
10. Waits appropriately for 10 min
11. Possesses and utilizes skills and strategies to manage emotions and sensory needs
12. Demonstrates problem solving
13. Safely engages in recreational or independent leisure activities for 15 min
14. Reads and writes functionally
15. Advocates for themself effectively

These IEP goals may at first glance appear to be small steps when trying to imagine a larger outcome. When developing goals related to the essential skills, it is often helpful to consider what opportunities are being presented to the student in order to practice this skill. For example, if a non-verbal student has a goal of requesting the use of the restroom consistently, but has not yet mastered keeping their augmentative and alternative control (AAC) or voice output device with them, it will be nearly impossible for them to master requesting the restroom using this method. In this example, the goal should be adjusted to teach the student how to request the restroom using multi-modal communication (e.g. using sign language, carrying a picture icon, having a picture icon available, gesturing, etc.) or wait on the requesting goal and use the time to focus on getting the student to take more ownership of the device across multiple settings and environments.

The aim of the educational team then, is to treat the process of transition planning as an ongoing conversation with the expectation that it will shift and get readjusted with each new development. All children grow and develop in unexpected ways over the course of adolescence. Autistic children are no different. If we are tasked with mapping out a plan, establishing goals, and creating innovative supports and accommodations to meet the unique needs of an autistic child, the plan cannot be rigid. The map must then be fluid and open to adjustment, and so must the team who draws the map.

5.5 Using Assessments to Develop Strong Goals

In order to develop the Individualized Education Plan (IEP) in the most informed manner, the educational team must conduct a series of researched-based, norm-referenced assessments. This is required by law for a child's initial IEP and at least every three years thereafter. There is a wealth of assessments that have been developed over the years that teachers and therapists can conduct to obtain the necessary information that identifies a child's strengths and significant areas of deficit that will help with establishing goals. Key areas assessed are: Academics, Functional Performance, Cognitive Functioning, Communication Status, Health, Hearing Vision, Motor Abilities, and Social-Emotional Status. When developing the transition plan and determining necessary instructional supports it is important to use assessments and educational models that target critical areas of functional life skills with an emphasis on an individual's knowledge, skills, and social communication abilities.

"The Taxonomy for Transition Programming 2.0" (Kohler et al. 2016), is an example of a model for planning, organizing, and evaluating transition education services and programs. This model focuses on five primary practice categories that have proven to be predictors of post-secondary success: Student-Focused Planning, Student Development, Interagency Collaboration, Family Engagement, and Program Structure. For teachers to be prepared to implement secondary transition evidence-based practices and predictors of post-school success teacher education programs must include these essential evidence-based components throughout a course of study (Morningstar and Mazzotti 2014). Extensive research shows that the taxonomy area of student development includes assessing and teaching functional, academic, social, and vocational skills to ensure that students are fully prepared for post-school life (Kohler et al. 2016). Formal and informal assessment data should be conducted to gather data that are used to drive instruction and assist in overcoming deficiencies as they are identified. Teachers should be prepared to teach and provide training related to independent living, community participation, employment skills, work-based experiences, academics, and self-determination.

The Community-Based Skills Assessment (CSA) is another tool that can be used to assist educators and families with the development of a personalized transition plan (Autism Speaks 2021). The CSA tool was developed for Autism Speaks in collaboration with Virginia Commonwealth University's Rehabilitation Research and Training Center. This assessment was designed to help parents and professionals assess the current skill levels and abilities of autistic individuals beginning at age 12 and continuing into adulthood in order to develop a comprehensive plan. The purpose is to assist teams in identifying areas of instructional priority for the individual. The creators of the CSA also state that while employment support needs of individuals are addressed through community-based internships and work experiences through school, this is the first tool to assess needs in the area of community-based living from transportation to financial management to peer relationships and more. For more information CSA tool visit https://www.autismspeaks.org/tool-kit/community-based-skills-assessment.

5.6 Exploring and Creating Options

Outside of building the transition plan and working with the educational team to create goals that match the projected outcomes for the student, experiential research by the parent(s) or supporting is needed. For many autistic students finding adult services and opportunities that match their specific combination of skills, interests, and support level is challenging. Additionally, depending on the district or geographic area where the student resides, the options may be limited or unclear.

In many districts and educational programs, a person or position is tasked with helping the student and family learn about and decide on what options are available in the community. This position, often the transition teacher, social worker, or a transition coordinator, is a great resource in terms of learning about the transition planning process, area agencies and options, and helping to make connections with community resource contacts that can assist in the transition process. However, these positions and the people in them should not be seen as the *only* way that a student is going to gain access to their next program or placement. Much of the exploration and especially the decision making should come from the family. Additionally, if a student is in an alternative program that is outside of their home district and community, then the options may be limited to the area of the school, rather than the community in which they reside. If the goal is for the student to have their post-secondary experience occur in an area that is closer to the family residence, then this should be another consideration for exploring options as early as possible in order to understand and plan for all of the variables.

As autism has been increasing in diagnosis numbers (CDC 2019) and increasing awareness in educational communities and national conversations has continued, more programs and options are being developed for autistic adults. Across the spectrum, agencies and companies are pushing old assumptions to create new and more dynamic programming that is inclusive of rather than just specific to autistic adults. Much of this growth has happened not in isolation or by accident. It has come from parents and caregivers who have advocated for the specific financial, geographic, support, and interest level needs of their children. This has inspired agencies and community programs to reach outside of the standard and invest in creating more diverse and relevant options (See Weitzberg, Chapter 5). The investigation of existing options and programs, along with the potential ability to influence the development of new options, will enhance the likelihood that the transition plan and IEP goals that the student has been working on will have an outcome that matches the hopes and efforts of the student and educational team.

Sam

At 16 Sam was a seemingly happy student enrolled in a therapeutic day school that was an out-placement from his assigned public school. Sam was diagnosed on the spectrum very early in his toddler years and had received special education services, including intensive speech services, since his diagnosis.

Sam is non-verbal, had difficulty staying with a group and would often wander off, with little awareness of his surroundings or safety. Sam needed full assistance with self-care including obtaining food, toileting, and communicating his immediate needs or wants.

Two specific educational goals that his school team focused on were:

- Staying with a small group
- Increasing functional communication, with the use of a generalizable support/device.

For Sam, over time during his high school years, he showed marked improvement in his ability to stay with a small group with reduced prompting and staff guidance. This was considered an educational success by his team. The educational goal that remained a challenge both in terms of progress, but also in considering options for adult placement, was finding and teaching a functional way for him to communicate his needs throughout the day. Over the years Sam had been exposed to a variety of communication systems. The style that was in use at the time of Sam's transition was a hip talker where the most consistent requests were placed on a voice output device that was attached like a belt around his waist. In this manner, Sam would not need to be responsible for carrying the device, which had proven to be a difficulty, but could be prompted by staff to point or press the device when seeking items as he wanted. At the time of his transition this was still an emerging skill.

Sam had very informed and active parents. They had been researching potential adult placements and options for Sam since he first entered late elementary school. They knew early on that they wanted to find an adult day program that could offer one-to-one support for Sam and was connected to a residential program. They were not certain that they wanted Sam to move out of their home right away, but did know that that was a long-term plan that made sense for their family.

The family was able to get Sam on the waitlist for state funding when he was just nine and began visiting and touring area adult day programs when Sam first entered high school. They initially were planning to have Sam complete both his high school and transition school years (through the end of his 21st birthday) with his school placement; however, Sam's name was pulled to receive state funding for residential and day programming during his last year in high school. Simultaneously, one of the adult day programs they had been working with had an opening in both their residential and day programs. The family, who had been active in the process and clear in their plans for Sam's exit, were able to make a quick decision and decided to end his school career early and have him not continue on to the transition program.

The agency they went with was able to assist them in completing the state paperwork to receive funding for a one-to-one placement. The family knew that this was rare in the adult program field and made the decision for Sam to leave school and move out quicker than they were originally planning because they saw it as an opportunity that matched with their long term goals for Sam. Sam was a better candidate for the program because, though he was still requiring a one-to-one staff, he was able to stay with the group more consistently and had a communication system that allowed for increased skill development and was something that was clear enough for the new placement's team to learn and incorporate into their environment.

The timeline for the transition was faster than originally expected but matched the needs of Sam and the family. The educational skills worked on during Sam's high school years increased his eligibility for the associated program. This transition, which involved parents that were strong researchers and advocates, an educational team that recognized the importance of transferable skills and supports, and an accepting agency that was willing to work with the family for appropriate state funding support, made this transition a success.

5.7 Determining 'Success'

Defining success in adulthood for any person making the journey from adolescence does not have a clear end point. For most, adulthood is a long and continual development of skills and experiences that lasts beyond the exit from secondary education. This is not untrue for an autistic person. Due to the broad nature of autism itself and the evolution of an individual's personhood into their twenties and beyond, the definition of success is as individualized as the person themselves.

For many students and families, success is defined by having a plan for post-secondary life that is attainable, meets the student where they are at academically and socially, and accurately connects the skills and talents of the student with opportunities for continued engagement, learning, and community connection. The time during the transition years often involves families and students adapting their perspective on what will be a successful outcome. Part of that determination is accomplished by the family and student researching and exploring what options are truly available in their geographic area and community for an autistic adult. Below is a case study that highlights a student and family's journey in that process and has outcomes that, for these individuals and their families, equate to a successful transition plan and outcome, even if it did not follow the original transition plan expectations.

Jerry

Jerry attended a typical public school in a self-contained classroom from early elementary through the end of his transition years. Jerry is nonverbal but is able to communicate his basic wants and needs through spelling out words and phrases on his communication device. Jerry uses software that is enabled onto an Android device so that it can fit in his pocket and he can pull it out when needed. The software allows for typing in manually, but also has predicting text to prompt familiar word use. Jerry is independent in his toileting needs, can complete concrete multi-step familiar tasks, and is able to stay with a group when asked.

During his time in high school and transition, his educational team focused on three specific educational goals related to his transition planning:

- Increase independent communication for wants and needs
- Increase ability to perform complex multi-step familiar tasks
- Decrease periods and intensity of anxiety or frustration

During the transition period out of school, Jerry's mother, Sue, was very active with the educational team and advocated for many of the supports and opportunities that had been made available to Jerry while in school to carry over to him once he exited. Sue worked with the school district so that Jerry could keep his communication device once he was done with school. This saved the family on cost and made the transition easy for Jerry's consistent communication method.

Sue worked with the transition team during Jerry's four years in the program to set up community volunteer opportunities that could continue outside of the school connection. Sue investigated several options for hiring a staff to work with Jerry at a variety of community sites so that he would continue to be supported and he would have guidance that was from other adults besides his mom. Sue met with the educational team to learn about the strategies that the school team used for when Jerry became anxious or frustrated so that she could ensure that she was using the same strategies at home but also be able to teach any new staff that Jerry would work with into his adulthood.

For the first few years after exiting his transition program, Jerry had a full weekly schedule that included one recurring paid position for two hours a week at a local restaurant rolling silverware, volunteering for two, 2-hour shifts at his local church, taking part in a therapeutic riding program, and going out for community trips with a staff one to two days per week. This schedule offered a variety of interactions, community connections, and highlighted several of the strong vocational skills that Jerry had developed over his years in school.

After a few years of this schedule, however, Jerry's family began to worry that he was too isolated. All of his experiences were happening in a one on one setting. The volunteering was at the church but was mostly interacting with his support staff. The riding was at a riding center but was primarily interacting with the instructor, and no other riders. Sue and her husband also worried that as both they and Jerry got older, the need to be connected to an agency would increase as they were less able to plan for and manage all of Jerry's placements and staffing. Jerry was lucky that Sue was such a strong advocate and had the time, resources, and ability to construct such a full schedule that built on Jerry's skills and interests. Sue recognized this as well and worried that it would be harder for him to go to a more group setting the longer he was away from peers or in situations where he had to use other skills to navigate interpersonal dynamics and unexpected situations.

When Jerry was in his mid-twenties, the family enrolled Jerry in an adult day program for one day a week. When in the day program, Jerry was able to complete a lot of the concrete tasks and activities that the new team presented to him. He was reliant on staff to prompt him to use his device for familiar wants and needs, such as asking for his snack or a glass of water. He would often wait and appear anxious, by rocking from side to side, until a staff acknowledged that it appeared like he needed something. Then Jerry would gesture to an area and staff would redirect him to use his device to request the item.

One challenge that Jerry had when in his school setting that began to change when in the adult day program was that he was initially very rigid about the timing of his schedule. If his daily schedule said that he was supposed to go on a community outing at 12:30 and the group was delayed, Jerry would become anxious and at times have heightened behaviors such as biting his fingers or hitting his hands to his head.

His awareness of time and its relationship to a schedule was also a strength at times rather than a hindrance and because of this was reinforced in the years when he was working with a one-to-one staff at volunteer sites. In that setting, Jerry had a written schedule, and when the time changed or he completed the stated number of items, he would move on to the next task with relative independence. When starting the adult day program, he found that what was once a skill often became a hindrance. In the adult day setting, there were many times that the group was not able to exit the building to start the outing at the exact minute that was listed on the schedule or an activity would be presented that was not as concrete and so would not be correlated with a quantity of steps. For example, in his volunteer settings Jerry would bag donated items for the church. The items were laid out in themed groups, in an assembly line fashion, and there was a clear order and quantity to follow. In the adult day program, there would be at times, tasks like this, and those remained the most familiar and easiest for Jerry to complete. However, there were also activities, like a music group, where Jerry was expected to wait between turns or to improvise the use of a musical instrument. In these instances, the expectations could not be laid out in a timeline or in relation to quantity quite as easily.

Initially, Jerry had some frustration and anxiety related to these changes. Additionally, the adult day program was louder and less predictable than the quietness of the church or equestrian program. During these periods, Jerry's anxiety and frustration would increase, and so would his negative behaviors related to these emotions. Jerry had periods of increased finger biting (his own), hitting his hands to his head, and clear looks of worry and anxiety. The staff at the adult day program worked with his mom and with their team to write out expectations more clearly for Jerry as well as encouraged Jerry to advocate if he needed a break. They showed him spaces that he could go if it was too noisy or he wanted a break from the activity. They continued to remind him that those were options and that with his communication device he could advocate independently during those times.

Over time, Jerry was able to get more comfortable with the noisiness and less predictable nature of the adult day program. His flexibility, self advocacy, and expressive communication skills expanded. His parents increased his days of attendance to three times a week. This way they were able to keep to his schedule of one day a week of therapeutic riding, one day a week of outside volunteering, and three days, where he could be with peers, continue to practice skills, and where his family did not have to plan for all of the activities of the day.

Jerry's family plans for this to be the schedule he maintains for several years, but anticipates that over the next decade it will likely change again as Jerry's and the family's needs evolve. The educational skills that Jerry's school team worked on with him served him well for his initial one-on-one placements post transition, and while they have been slightly altered in a new setting and continue to be addressed, they are still the foundational skills that are helping him to be successful in a combination of individual and group settings.

5.8 Where Do We Go from Here?

Parents, educators, and autistic individuals are already navigating the complex day-to-day challenges that life on the spectrum can present. They are doing this while also embracing what can be delightfully surprising interactions and perspectives that autistic people bring into the world and to the people that love and support them. For a student who finds the deepest satisfaction in scripting the entire dialogue from the movie *Cars 2* at the age of 18 in the middle of dinner every night, or has difficulty navigating the nuance of the social etiquette expectations of the high school hallway and thus needs an aide to assist with the walk between classes, those challenges can feel immediate and daunting. The energy required to address them and put supports in place to decrease the related impulses and anxieties that can take away from the positive and pleasurable sides of life on the spectrum takes daily effort from the entire educational team, including the student. For autistic students, this type of challenge does not come in isolation, but rather as a package containing other physiological, social, and often cognitive needs. To add planning for adulthood as well as options that are truly practical and accessible for autistic adults, can make this topic feel like a colossal task for all involved.

The recommendation is not to view the educational components of the transition planning process as linear but instead as likely to weave in and out of successes and setbacks—not to expect transition planning to start at a set age after some random assigned 'other' tasks or goals have been met but to plan for it to be integrated into the ongoing conversation. Trust that it will come together bit by bit, with the collaboration of the many teachers, educators, caregivers, and community members invested in the student's progress. Trust that the student, when invited into the transition planning process, will give insight into what will be the most beneficial and successful next steps for their life. With intentional planning while still remaining open to adjustment as the student grows and changes, transition planning can become individualized, meaningful, and realistic. Most excitingly, with continued feedback and effort from the related stakeholders, society can expand to create more space and opportunities for autistic adults. A successful transition plan for an autistic adult has the potential not just to maximize the happiness, success, and purpose of that one person, but to positively impact the community as a whole.

5.9 Appendix 1: Page 2 of the Giant Steps PREP Packet

Transition Timeline Reference

Things to Consider and Address from Ages 14–22.

(Adapted from Chicago Public Schools' 'Transition Timeline and Planning' 2012).

14 Year Olds

- Attend transition nights within your school district to find out about transition programming and supports available.
- Identify personal learning styles and the necessary accommodations for successful learning and working.
- Increase your child's ability to communicate effectively about interests, preferences and needs.
- Help your child to learn to explain his/her own disability and the accommodations needed, as appropriate for your child.
- Investigate and explore assistive technology tools that can increase community involvement and employment opportunities.

- Broaden your child's experiences with community activities and build relationships in the community.
- Explore money management and identify needed skill area.
- Identify and begin learning skills necessary for independent living, as appropriate for your child.
- Learn and practice personal health care.
- Obtain functional vocational assessment.
- Discuss taxes and medical insurance and other benefits.
- Establish graduation date.
- Visit vocational, educational and residential options if appropriate.
- Write transition goals on IEP and invite service providers to IEP meeting.
- Review high school course of study and vocational options.

15 Year Olds

- Include adult service providers in transition planning meeting (i.e. PAS agency).
- Apply for SSI, public aid and general assistance.
- Implement guardianship, power of attorney, wills/trusts.
- Contact special needs coordinator at college, if appropriate.
- Register for selective service (males).
- Invite service providers to IEP meeting.
- Review high school course of study and vocational options.

16 Year Olds

- Provide opportunities for your child to learn and practice appropriate interpersonal, communication and social skills for different settings (employment, recreation, with peers, with family, etc.).
- Practice independent living skills (i.e. shopping, cooking, housekeeping, grooming, and budgeting).
- Apply for Medicaid, if appropriate.
- Obtain driver's license or state ID card.
- Pursue Adult Education.
- Development of an interagency agreement with local service providers.
- Systematic phase out of school supports and phase in of adult services.
- Invite service providers to IEP meetings.
- Review high school course of study and vocational options.

17 Year Olds

- Parental trainings and student training in lifelong planning (person-centered planning).
- Student participates and contributes to IEP development as appropriate.
- Explore community recreational and leisure interests.
- Discuss medical needs and related services.
- Consider need for independent living skills.
- Begin early career exploration.
- Consider options for summer programs.

- Write transition goals in the IEP.
- Invite service providers to IEP meeting.
- At evaluation/re-evaluation indicate the need for transition services.
- Include high school course of study in the IEP.

18 Year Olds

- Discuss SSI and SSWI (social security work incentives).
- Discuss funding sources for home services.
- Participate in interest/vocational inventory (self-directed search).
- Review future living options.
- Explore current and future living options.
- Consider referral to the Illinois Department of Human Services (DHS/DORS)
- Write transition goals in the IEP.
- Invite service providers to IEP meeting.
- Review high school course of study and vocational options.

19–21 Year Olds

- Participate in interest/vocational/engagement inventory (self-directed search).
- Discuss supported employment, job coaching, day programming
- Access job shadowing or volunteering.
- Consider work training, post-secondary education, day programming, or community engagement options
- Introduce to student if appropriate the concept of guardianship, power of attorney, wills/trusts.
- Write transition goals in the IEP.
- Invite service providers to IEP meeting.
- Review high school course of study and vocational options.
- Make referral to DORS.

*Be creative. Talk to other parents, get involved with agencies whom you support their service delivery or approach to meet the needs of the individuals they serve, and work collaboratively having many conversations to develop the best fit for your child for whatever services they need or options you want to see for them.

References

Anderson, K.A., C. Sosnowy, A. Kuo, and P.T. Shattuck. 2018. Transition of individuals with autism to adulthood: A review of qualitative studies. *Pediatrics* 141 (S4): S318–S327. https://doi.org/10.1542/peds.2016-4300I.

Autism Speaks. 2021. Autism statistics and facts. https://www.autismspeaks.org/autism-statistics. Accessed 20 Mar 2021.

Autism Speaks. 2021. Community-based Skills Assessment (CSA): Developing a personalized transition plan. https://www.autismspeaks.org/tool-kit/community-based-skills-assessment. Accessed 20 Mar 2021.

Centers for Disease Control and Prevention, Autism Spectrum Disorder. https://www.cdc.gov/ncbddd/autism. Accessed 20 Mar 2021.

Department of Education, Office of Special Education and Rehabilitative Services. 2017. A transition guide to postsecondary education and employment for students and youth with disabilities. https://www2.ed.gov/about/offices/list/osers/transition/products/postsecondary-transition-guide-2017.pdf?utm_content=&utm_medium=email&utm_name=&utm_s.

Individuals with Disabilities Education Act (IDEA). 2006 (US).

Kohler, P.D., J.E. Gothberg, C. Fowler, and J. Coyle. 2016. Taxonomy for transition programming 2.0: A model for planning, organizing, and evaluating transition education, services, and programs. Western Michigan University. https://transitionta.org/system/files/resourcetrees/Taxonomy_for_Transition_Programming_v2_508_.pdf?file=1&type=node&id=1727&force=.

Learning Disabilities Association of America. 2021. https://ldaamerica.org. Accessed 20 Mar 2021.

Morningstar, M., and V. Mazzotti. 2014. Teacher preparation to deliver evidence-based transition planning and services to youth with disabilities (Document No. IC-1). Retrieved from University of Florida, Collaboration for Effective Educator, Development, Accountability, and Reform Center. http://ceedar.education.ufl.edu/tools/innovation-configurations/.

Robison, J.E. 2018. Life, love, and happiness for autistic adults. *Psychology Today*. https://www.psychologytoday.com/us/blog/my-life-aspergers/201809/life-love-and-happiness-autistic-adults. Accessed 20 Mar 2021.

Wehman, P., M.D. Smith, and C. Schall. 2009. *Autism and the transition to adulthood: Success beyond the classroom*. Baltimore: Paul H. Brookes Pub. Co.U.S.

Chapter 6
Employment Issues Related to Transition: Lessons from Aspiritech

Moshe Weitzberg

Abstract This chapter outlines some of the benefits and challenges of employing autistic individuals based on the experiences of only one company. Potential employers should understand and expect that they certain accommodations will need to be made to successfully recruit, hire, and employ autistic individuals. The company described in this chapter, Aspiritech, employs more than 100 autistic adults, so we have encountered many issues over the years. Accommodations (if any) will vary in scale and degree depending upon the number of autistic individuals hired. As this chapter illustrates, there are countless benefits of employing autistic individuals, and autistic employees can be a tremendous asset to a workplace. We recognize that the information provided in this chapter and the company described reflect only a small subset of autistic individuals, however, even within that small subset, the range of supports needed vary from individual to individual.

6.1 Introduction

As the founders of Aspiritech, a quality assurance (QA) testing company that empowers autistic individuals to fulfill their potential through meaningful employment combined with social opportunity, we want to share our experience with those who are interested in, and could benefit from, hiring a group of capable yet underutilized individuals. We have found that autistic adults have many desirable characteristics, including reliability, honesty, incredible memory, attention to detail combined with strong logic and analytical and technical skills, making them important assets to the business community.

In this article, we outline some of the benefits and challenges of employing autistic individuals. Potential employers should understand and expect that they will need to make certain accommodations to successfully recruit, hire, and employ autistic individuals. Aspiritech employs more than 100 autistic adults, so we have encountered

M. Weitzberg (✉)
Aspiritech NFP, 319 Euclid Avenue, Highwood, IL 60040, USA
e-mail: moshe@aspiritech.org

N. Elster and K. Parsi (eds.), *Transitioning to Adulthood with Autism: Ethical, Legal and Social Issues*, The International Library of Bioethics 91,
https://doi.org/10.1007/978-3-030-91487-5_6

many issues over the years. Accommodations (if any) will vary in scale and degree depending upon the number of autistic individuals hired. As this article illustrates, there are countless benefits of employing autistic individuals, and autistic employees can be a tremendous asset to a workplace.

6.2 Background

In 2008, we heard about a Danish company called Specialisterne (the Specialists) who employed autistic adults (https://specialisterne.com/). Other similar companies emerged in Europe. We decided to try the concept in the United States.

The European model involved a lengthy screening and training process often funded by European governments. Most graduates of the European programs worked as consultants in the IT industry, complementing QA teams when companies experienced heavy workloads. The consultants worked in an inclusive environment and sometimes needed to move from one company to another. We were unable to duplicate this model since government support was not available. We eventually founded Aspiritech in 2008 as a not-for-profit entity with public donations as the main source of income. We opened Aspiritech as a not-for-profit outsourced QA company, supported by public donations with services provided entirely by autistic adults.

6.3 Beginning

In January 2010, we opened our first small office outside of Chicago in Highland Park, Illinois, without a single client on our roster. We focused on identifying clients who would be willing to try us out. Aspiritech needed to prove to the business community that autistic adults are able to provide exceptional QA services. Many volunteers helped us to acquire clients, and we slowly grew our business. For a few years, we only had a single project at a time, and there were days without client work; no companies were yet willing to trust their entire QA project to autistic adults.

Aspiritech's growth relied entirely on its reputation. It took approximately four years of very slow growth to get the business community to feel comfortable with Aspiritech, and only in 2014 did Aspiritech's client revenue exceed philanthropic support. Aspiritech started growing faster around this time because major news outlets started reporting on how some autistic adults have exceptional talents that meet business needs (Elejalde-Ruiz 2006). Some of these media outlets wrote about us and filmed our operations (Tynan 2014). Our clients started to give us more projects and responsibilities.

During the earlier difficult years, when growth was slow and business was scarce, we complemented analysts' time with social activities. Our current supportive and accommodating workspace started when there was very little work and we could pay close attention to the best environment for and needs of our employees. We quickly realized how important it was to provide social opportunities to fill the downtime. Understanding the unique needs of our analysts led us to create the Stepping Up and Out (SUO) program (explained later). Today, Aspiritech is known for its accommodating and supportive work environment that enables our talented analysts to perform their best work for our clients. Our first support specialist, Marc Lazar, was instrumental in creating an accommodating work environment, which we continue to develop and improve upon. Aspiritech currently employs a team of Employment Support Specialists who help facilitate special and individualized accommodations and after-work and weekend social activities.

Aspiritech is now a $5.5 million company providing very complex and critical QA services to multiple of client companies such as Zebra Technologies and JP Morgan Chase thanks to the operational staff that is more than 90% neurodivergent (with autism and additional related conditions such as OCD, ADHD, Tourette's). Ninety-two percent of our current revenue is derived from client services.

6.4 Onboarding and Interviewing

Most of our first analysts did not have any previous meaningful work experience of significant duration. Some had worked in the retail industry, doing work that was not commensurate with their skills, and some had moved from one job to another. Others had given up on securing employment and stayed at home. Some had never worked before. Our goal was to train and certify our new recruits as QA analysts and employ them on multiple projects.

When we first started interviewing potential analysts, we could tell that they had received training in "interview etiquette." They often shook hands very firmly, looked straight into our eyes and tried to look professional. Some applicants tried to "mask" the fact that they were on the autism spectrum (some had even been coached to do this), making attempts to act like neurotypicals. Many were terrified by the interview process and some asked to reschedule. Initially, we did not start with a phone interview, nor did we test applicants on their computer skills or conduct other screening tests to see if they were a good fit for the position. However, it did not take us long to change our methods. We learned to inform applicants about the interview process ahead of time to avoid surprising the candidate. If desired, potential analysts could bring a family member, job coach and/or their therapist to the interview. Not everyone did, but for some, it was very helpful. This minor change made a huge difference in the interview process. Today, we rarely allow a third person to be present during the interview process, but one of our Employment Support Staff sits in on the interview to help ease tension and create a more relaxing atmosphere. They intervene at the first sign of stress.

In those early years, we began each interview by asking about the applicant's time in school and college. We heard difficult stories about their experiences in middle and high school, including references to physical and verbal abuse and being excluded and undermined by other students, teachers and even family members. Some parents told us how their children refused to leave the car when they were driven to school in the morning. We also learned how brave they were to arrive to school each day and face a hostile environment. We heard about their many years of isolation; this was concerning since QA testing requires a strong degree of teamwork.

One of our first clients created chat rooms for children with disabilities where they could text, either in groups or individually. The client asked us to test the language filter that prevents "dirty" words or expressions. We had "fun" trying out every offensive expression that came to mind. Afterwards, our analysts told our client that for them the "F" word and other profanities did not impact them, whereas words such as "retard," "idiot," "stupid," "slow" or even "you do not understand" were devastating. It was hard for them to test these offensive words/expressions in the language filter. As a result, we started to emphasize the value of respect, and made every effort to prevent any insulting or disrespectful behavior toward each other and clients. Occasionally, we need to remind our clients that our analysts do not have proper understanding of social cues and they can say or hear things in unexpected ways.

6.5 Quality Assurance and Software Testing

Many facets are included under the umbrella of QA and software testing, including regression, acceptance, usability, functionality, integration testing and many more. The purpose of the profession is to provide a very high-quality product that is not only "bug free" but also easy to use and covers all functionalities. Aspiritech's objective is to help the client achieve a high-quality product by teaming up with the clients' developers and QA groups, not just pointing out bugs. The analyst is required to learn the methodology of creating test cases that cover all the functions and should be able to follow them again and again, each time that the developer makes changes, in order to verify that everything works as expected (this is known as regression testing). Some tasks may seem very repetitive to a neurotypical individual, but our employees usually enjoy finding seemingly small irregularities.

The analyst must become the Subject Matter Expert (SME) of the product, more so even than the developers themselves. The focus is not on what is the same but rather on what is different or unexpected. Being the SME helps the analyst to spot minor irregularities and suggest improvements. Aspiritech analysts are trained along this line.

Most people are not well suited to be QA and software analysts, regardless of their talent and IT knowledge, but a large percentage of autistic adults thrive in these roles. The work requires continual focus, and for many it is tedious, exhausting and often under-appreciated. Yet, in the age of instant reviews and product refunds, QA work is becoming a critical need for clients.

6.6 Training

Aspiritech rarely hires individuals with previous experience in the QA arena. This ensures that new applicants adapt to the Aspiritech style and culture while learning the software testing and QA craft. Aspiritech provides a comprehensive paid (via stipend) training to applicants, typically in groups of 10–12. The applicants who successfully complete the training are offered positions. QA work is very unique and requires a certain type of personality to really enjoy and succeed at it over the long run. For instance, one of our employees, before arriving at Aspiritech, had spent a good deal of time pointing out typos in restaurant menus, out of a genuine desire for the restaurant to improve its copy-editing; this employee is now a lead on the largest project at Aspiritech. The training consists of two parts: a one-week, hands-on classroom instruction on the basics of software testing and on our QA philosophy of working alongside the developers to bring a quality product to the market, followed by at least two weeks of applying what has been learned working alongside staff on client work.

During the first week, interviewees are actively exposed to the basic elements of software testing via hands-on practice. They follow test cases (a written script for manual testing), create test cases, and then review each other's work to learn how to identify, investigate and document defects. This part requires very intensive guidance, focus and supervision. We assign a job coach to every two to three applicants and at least one employment support specialist for the entire training group. The applicants get to know what Aspiritech is all about and gain a feel for the core values of the company. During the first week, most of the applicants are able to determine if this is the right job for them, and we get to know them and how they work in a team environment. Typically, one to three applicants leave the training at this point, usually because they do not see themselves doing QA work for a very long time. Occasionally, we tell applicants that they are not a good fit for the job.

The second part of the training takes place in smaller groups of three to four and lasts at least two weeks. Trainees are often embedded with our analysts and perform work comparable to client work that we have already completed (our clients embrace this method since it is a way to train more analysts on their applications without costing them a dime). The trainees are mentored by our job coaches and analysts and have the opportunity to get to know the managers and the company structure.

The training process is seemingly costly, but the reward is having new hires who are competent, more likely to remain with the company, and capable of providing quality, high-value services to our clients. We pay our trainees a stipend during the training process and we pay the coaches and mentors for their time with the trainees; this strategy helps us determine what kind of work is the best fit for each applicant and what accommodations he or she might need. Once applicants successfully complete both parts of the training and come onboard as employees, they are able to provide quality work to our clients almost immediately. At the moment, we do not provide training as a stand-alone service for revenue.

The purpose of this training model is to identify talented autistic adults who can be very productive in the QA field, appear to enjoy this type of work and are interested in developing a vocation. Such talent is very difficult to find among any group. When this is done successfully, the results are satisfied clients who recommend our work to others, respect neurodiversity and the strengths of the autism community, and find joy in helping an under-appreciated segment of our population.

6.7 Work Routine

Many of our analysts are not able to work longer than four hours/day when they are first hired. This is similar to what we learned from a few European companies that specialize in work with autistic adults. Aspiritech invites people to work on a regular basis according to their requests (part of our accommodation policy). After several months, many analysts are able to increase their workday to 6+ hours/day; consistent scheduling according to the analyst's request is a key to achieving this goal. We also see a notable frequency of analysts who give last-minute notice that they are unable to show up for work. This is usually due to genuine medical issues related to their comorbid conditions such as headaches, migraines, stomach discomforts, fatigue or pain. We believe most of these are not "excuses;" these are real issues. With proper support, work attendance improves dramatically. In anticipation of unpredictable attendance, we try to have enough analysts scheduled to cover for each other. To an outsider, such inconsistency would seem to be unacceptable, but in our experience, it rarely is. Despite the inconvenience this causes, our analysts bring tremendous value to our clients and, therefore, these incidents are tolerated and typically become scarcer over time (there are exceptions, of course). Employers who want to benefit from the talent that autistic adults can bring to the workplace need to take these issues into account and work with the analyst to minimize inconsistency in attendance.

The IT industry, and especially service-provider companies such as Aspiritech, do not have uniform workloads. There are times when the workload is very light while at other times the pressure to complete a project by a specific date is great, and consequently overtime and weekend work are required. Autistic individuals do not do well when the workload is inconsistent and especially when it is low. This is when our support staff are critical to Aspiritech's operations. We provide meaningful activities such as cross-training, certifications, IT courses and other related tasks to fill in workflow gaps and enable analysts to develop their skills and be able to move to other projects that require fortification.

Some of our clients rely on the holiday season to generate the bulk of their income. For these clients, the pre-holiday time is critical and the race to provide quality applications or devices in time for the Thanksgiving/Christmas sales creates a huge pressure on our employees. Review of bugs is more frequent, deadlines are shorter and we often need to work overtime and weekends to meet the goals. Such stressful weeks can cause issues that our support staff is usually able to handle. It is often the "down time" after the product's release that is more stressful. Less work often results in employees who are anxious, fearful of losing their jobs, and perhaps even feeling a bit empty inside. These situations place a tremendous strain on the time of our Employment Support Specialists who must ramp up the frequency of their meetings with our analysts to help address their increased anxieties. Acknowledging this fluctuating workload, learning new skills by cross-training on other projects and mentoring others who want to learn can help to alleviate the problem. Yet when the work finally begins again, it can be another slight challenge to get back into the work routine.

6.8 Support

The ability to manage an unpredictable work routine requires complex executive functioning skills of observing, organizing and planning what needs to be done. Autistic individuals often have difficulties with communication and social interactions and sensory/repetitive interests and behaviors. These issues can negatively impact an individual's likelihood of finding a job or even getting through the first step of the job search. While these are common characteristics of autism, it is important to remember that each person has a unique set of skills, challenges and personal traits. Support staff and our supportive environment are key to Aspiritech's success. Aspiritech goes to great lengths to support autistic employees. Any one of the many possible accommodations we offer may be needed only for very few individuals or often for only one person. If a person is capable of doing the work and enjoys it, we will try to provide reasonable accommodations. Employers interested in employing autistic individuals can benefit by hiring a few capable yet underutilized individuals and may not need to provide nearly as many accommodations as we do. For the record, the majority of our analysts do not need accommodations; however, those who can benefit from accommodations are provided with accommodations tailored to their own needs. Often, these are minor considerations. Our support addresses the following general issues:

1. Environment to address sensory tolerances
2. Distractions
3. Changes
4. Understanding job directions by using written instructions
5. Communication
6. Social opportunities, after-work activities.

6.9 Sensory Issues

Many autistic adults have a certain degree of sensory intolerance. For the majority, it has to do with sound and/or light. These issues can manifest themselves not only in different ways but can also be more acute on different days and/or times of the day. Aspiritech installed expensive LED light fixtures to simulate natural light and avoid flickering. We also built several sensory break rooms where employees can decompress, dim the lights, put on a weighted vest, use fidget instruments, lie down and relax, or even take a short nap. These rooms are often in use, though usually only for relatively short periods.

Sensitivity to sound is more common in autistic individuals and, in most cases, easy to address by providing noise-canceling headphones. In rare cases, certain sounds can cause an intense reaction (such as leaving the workplace). We observed intolerance to loud voices, laughter, the clicking sound of keyboards and the squashing of candy wrappers. Aspiritech has two kitchens: a small one is designated as the quiet kitchen and the need for silence is respected there, while the larger (and more popular) kitchen is a conversational space. The conversational kitchen is equipped with a volume meter which turns red when the conversation becomes too loud; this device helps staff to self-monitor.

We have not observed extreme intolerance to smell, but our outside consultant strongly suggested that employees not wear strong perfumes and so far everyone has respected this mandate. Construction/chemical smells in a building could trigger some unusual reactions. Additionally, we found that employees who had candles or oil for aromatherapy were asked by their colleagues to stop using those materials.

6.10 Distractions

Among the most disruptive issues for some of our autistic analysts are distractions caused by mobile devices and websites such as social media (especially Facebook), YouTube, blogs, games, and emails. Many QA tests require waiting for a period of time—for example, when testing if an application goes to "sleep" or turns itself off properly. During such periods, some analysts will start using their phones or other mobile devices to visit their favorite websites. Often they become immersed in their devices and "forget" everything. Before starting work at Aspiritech, many employees spent their entire day in front of a game console, computer or mobile device. Their familiarity with many aspects of technology is a huge asset. However, the addictive nature of some sites can affect employees' productivity and ability to spot bugs. Our support staff have found several solutions for these issues, each customized to the individual. For instance, some employees are provided regular short breaks to clock out and spend time on their favorite websites; they use a stopwatch to remind themselves to clock back in again after the specified amount of time. In some cases, the analysts themselves ask the support team to keep their personal phone and get it back at lunch and before leaving work.

Most analysts, however, learn within a short time to focus on the tasks at hand and to abandon their phones during work time. When we notice analysts spending more time on their phones, it is often a sign of anxiety or another issue that requires support intervention.

6.11 Changes

The only constant in today's workplace is change; the ability to continually adapt is crucial. Continued support tailored to an individual's personality and work style needs to be implemented and refined as needed. Change is one of the most difficult factors for many autistic people to handle. Often, minor changes are much more difficult than major ones. One of our high-performing analysts, who is uncommonly at ease transitioning between projects, was sitting alone in a corner and expressed distress about being isolated. When we moved the analyst (after careful preparation) between two colleagues only a few feet away, the change overwhelmed the employee, who had to go home. It took this employee a few days to recuperate and return to work.

It is common for autistic individuals to have multiple diagnoses. Some are physical (such as fine and gross motor skills) or mental health issues (ADHD, OCD, anxiety). Many of these are not manifested during a regular work routine but can come to light when change occurs. For example, one of our analysts needed to change workstations and was annoyed not to find his marked mouse, although there were others available that looked the same. Our support team is trained to quickly address and resolve these issues.

6.12 Understanding Job Directions by Using Written Instructions

Many of our analysts do not process verbal instructions as well as written ones. Written instructions help analysts maintain focus and complete their tasks. This is actually a benefit for QA work since they carefully read manuals and requirements and can easily spot discrepancies within applications. A company like Aspiritech provides QA testing to many industries. Analysts need to become familiar with two or three different projects and be ready to swap between them and change their focus. The support team makes sure that analysts have clear written instructions to avoid surprises and allow for smooth transitions between projects.

6.13 Communication

A major hurdle often overlooked are communication difficulties noted in the interview process. These issues continue in employees' daily work with colleagues and supervisors. Autistic individuals often have difficulty reading social cues and figuring out implied meanings, which can result in anxiety and frustration. Clear support and feedback are needed to address such issues, and it is crucial that supervisors and peers work to provide this feedback from a position of cooperation and understanding. A lifetime of feeling abused, disregarded, isolated and excluded can contribute to anxieties. The most important role of the support team is to meet with analysts who so choose (most of them do) on a regular basis and as needed. The goal of the support is to help analysts be productive by helping them emotionally and providing coping mechanisms/suggestions. When an analyst starts to have problems related to productivity (absences and the like) the supervisor contacts the assigned support team member before talking to the analyst. In rare cases and by required signed permission of the analyst, the support staff consults with the employee's personal therapist or family member(s). Often, a short communication with the family therapist can help the analyst become productive again.

In general, family members are very anxious to know how their relative is doing and whether they are adapting to work. However, this is confidential information that we cannot provide. Aspiritech's goal is to help our staff grow in independence; family involvement is only initiated if there is a real need (and, of course, with signed consent from the employee).

6.14 Lunch Discussions

Every two weeks, analysts who so wish meet for lunch group discussions. Attendance is not required and is at the sole discretion of each individual. The topics are chosen by our analysts and conversation is facilitated by one or two of the Employment Support Specialists. The lunch discussions last 45–60 minutes. In general, management is not invited to these sessions, and the support representative is there to answer questions, provide information and references and ensure that the group remains focused on the topic. The lunch discussions are a safe space for analysts to share their personal experiences of coping with certain situations. When a topic is very popular, the group goes to a nearby restaurant with a private room, and the discussion can continue during the next meeting. Here are examples of past topics:

- Professional networking
- Depression and anxiety
- Independent living
- Relationships and dating
- Making friends/socializing
- Hobbies and interests.

6.15 Social Opportunities and After-Work Activities

Aspiritech provides two categories of after-work and weekend activities. The first type of activity occurs during the workday. The analysts have initiated several "clubs" that they also manage, such as: Game Clubs, Book Club, Movie Club, Coding Club, and more. The opportunity to plan social activities allows our analysts to share their interests, convince others to join in, maintain quality relationships and learn how to involve members so that the activity will not subside. The second category of activity, Stepping Up and Out (SUO) , is initiated and managed by Aspiritech. SUO is typically held on Sundays for five hours, but sometimes it is extended to other days (for example, if Aspiritech obtains tickets to popular events). This program is managed by an outside professional, is financed entirely by donations and is open to any autistic individual, not only Aspiritech employees. The SUO activity changes each week. It can be improvisation by a trained actor, going to the movies, live theater, music and sporting events, museums, playing sports such as basketball or bowling, and more. These events allow Aspiritech analysts to forge a community, building friendships and even romantic relationships. The support, kindness and sensitivity of our analysts toward each other helps to make these events very successful. Together with their daily work, these events are truly life-changing.

6.16 Sexual Orientation

More than 10% of our analysts are members of the LGBTQ community. At least half of them self-disclosed their gender and/or sexual identity after being at Aspiritech for at least six months. Gay Pride month was celebrated in the office for the first time in 2019 and a group of employees attended the annual Gay Pride parade together. Please see Kahn, Chap. 3 for more information about LGBTQ and autistic individuals.

6.17 Summary

Aspiritech created a successful quality assurance business where the workforce is almost entirely comprised of autistic adults. The Aspiritech model trains the candidates and later provides internationally recognized certification. Aspiritech's standalone model operates in the same way as a "typical" work environment but with an emphasis on training and strong employment support. The goal of the support is to guide our analysts to become independent and minimize their reliance on others. The support team is not involved in the QA operations. Aspiritech leadership is mostly grown internally; the majority of the project leads began as analysts. Leads and analysts communicate directly with the clients and work independently. Daily interaction with the client, verbally or written, is the window where our analysts are communicating as equals with the neurotypical (aka inclusive) world. Our clients "forget" that they are dealing with autistic individuals and are happy to discuss issues and suggestions with our analysts. Almost all the clients visit Aspiritech on a regular basis (even from other states) and occasionally we visit them. During these meetings, we discuss the major issues, obstacles, suggestions and plans for the future. We believe that our model is a very effective way for our analysts to be able to succeed in a competitive environment in the future, if they so desire.

At the end of the day, it is a win-win-win situation:

Win: Autistic analysts create a social circle, learn a profession and feel accomplished at work.
Win: Society and families get support exclusively caring for their relatives.
Win: The business community benefits from world-class quality assurance and software testing services.

Acknowledgements I would like to thank all the people that helped and advised on this chapter: Ann Brownell, our CTO; Christian Durantes, Reanin Stone and Bonny Goldin, our support staff; Linda Hoeck our consultant; and Kelsey Schagemann who edited the manuscript. Special thanks to Lauren Birnhak and Michael Ashburne, our project leads who read and remarked on each topic.

Special thanks to my wife Brenda Weitzberg, whose initiative and vision of creating Aspiritech transformed so many lives, including mine. You brought special meaning to my life!

References

Elejalde-Ruiz, A. 2006. 'It's changed his view of life': Companies find hiring autistic employees has vast benefits. *Chicago Tribune.* https://www.chicagotribune.com/business/ct-autism-workplace-hart-schaffner-marx-0612-biz-20160610-story.html. Accessed 2 Apr 2021

Tynan, D. (2014). Eight things you ought to know about autism (and might not). *Yahoo.* https://finance.yahoo.com/news/eight-things-you-ought-to-know-about-autism-but-might-84070057936.html. Accessed 2 Apr 2021

Chapter 7
Driving/Transportation and Transition

Haley J. Bishop, Allison E. Curry, and Benjamin E. Yerys

Abstract Compared to people with access to reliable means of transportation, individuals with transportation barriers are more likely to have chronic diseases or other health problems—making it especially important for these individuals to attend regular health appointments and adhere to their medications. In this chapter, we will discuss transportation in the context of both independent driving and other forms of transportation in the autistic population. For autistic drivers, we examine the challenges to independent driving and the learning-to-drive process, as well as recommendations for caregivers and programs aimed at addressing these challenges. Finally, other forms of independent mobility available to the autistic population will be reviewed. In sum, finding effective ways to improve the transportation ability of autistic individuals as they transition to adulthood is critical given its effect on short- and long-term quality of life and well-being.

7.1 Importance of Transportation for Adulthood

Access to reliable means of transportation is often overlooked as an important determinant of various social, health, and economic outcomes in an individual's life. People without access to transportation feel thwarted from participating in activities that affect their quality of life and feel socially excluded and isolated (Lucas and Currie 2012). Additionally, transportation barriers are especially common for marginalized populations, including people living in poverty or with physical and developmental disabilities (Danziger 1999; Lubin 2012). The 2017 Interagency Autism Coordinating Committee emphasized the urgent need for services that improve the functioning and quality of life of autistic individuals as they transition from adolescence to adulthood (Interagency Autism Coordinating Committee 2017), which is particularly challenging for them and their families. Many services

H. J. Bishop · A. E. Curry (✉) · B. E. Yerys
Center for Injury Research and Prevention at CHOP, 2716 South Street 13th Floor, Philadelphia, PA 19146, USA
e-mail: currya@email.chop.edu

N. Elster and K. Parsi (eds.), *Transitioning to Adulthood with Autism: Ethical, Legal and Social Issues*, The International Library of Bioethics 91,
https://doi.org/10.1007/978-3-030-91487-5_7

once received through special education are no longer available after age 21 in most states (some end at 22) and adult services are difficult to access (Taylor and Henninger 2015). A national survey reported that more than 1 in 3 autistic individuals did not transition to employment or education after high school, more than 1 in 4 were socially isolated, and about 1 in 3 had no community participation in the past year (Roux et al. 2015). These missed opportunities can have substantial long-term negative consequences on independence and quality of life (Geller and Greenberg 2009). Young autistic individuals commonly report feeling trapped at home and unable to work because of transportation issues. In fact, in a 2009 New Jersey state-wide survey, autistic individuals and their caretakers noted transportation as a significant obstacle to participation in work (50.9%) and non-work (48.0%) activities, leaving the population heavily reliant (81.6%) on friends and families to meet transportation needs (Feeley 2010). Transportation is also highly indicative of an individual's level of independence, which is itself an important factor of social, health, and economic success (Dickerson et al. 2007; Huang et al. 2012). With respect to health outcomes, transportation barriers may also impact a person's ability to regularly attend health care appointments and travel to pharmacies, resulting in poor health and medication adherence (Syed et al. 2013). This is especially concerning as researchers have found that compared to people with access to reliable means of transportation, individuals with transportation barriers are more likely to have chronic diseases or other health problems—making it especially important for these individuals to attend regular health appointments and adhere to their medications (Syed et al. 2013; Wallace et al. 2005). In sum, finding effective ways to improve the transportation ability of autistic individuals as they transition to adulthood is critical given its effect on short- and long-term quality of life and well-being.

In this chapter, we will discuss transportation in the context of both independent driving and other forms of transportation in the autistic population. For autistic drivers, we will examine the challenges to independent driving and the learning-to-drive process, as well as recommendations for caregivers and programs that address these challenges. Finally, other forms of independent mobility available to the autistic population will be reviewed.

7.2 Independent Driving

An important milestone that typically occurs during adolescence is obtaining a driver's license. Licensure increases adolescents' mobility by enabling independent travel to places of employment, school, and social activities (Winston and Senerrick 2006). For children diagnosed on the autism spectrum without an intellectual disability (ID)[1] in the early 2000s, who are approaching driving age, the decision to drive and the challenges that will accompany this task are nearing quickly (Centers

[1] Hereafter 'autism' or 'autism spectrum' will refer to subgroup of autistic individuals without intellectual disability.

for Disease Control and Prevention 2018). In a cohort of autistic teens in New Jersey born in 1987–1995, 1 in 3 acquired a driver's license by age 21 and nearly 90% of those who acquired a permit went on to get licensed within two years—only slightly lower than adolescents without Autism Spectrum Disorder (ASD) (98%) (Curry et al. 2017). These results suggest that a substantial proportion of autistic adolescents do get licensed and that license-related decisions are primarily made prior to the teen ever getting behind the wheel.

Finding a balance between autonomy and safety is likely to be a particularly sensitive task for families of autistic adolescents—and one that may impact the decision to pursue licensure. By definition, autistic individuals typically have deficits in skills known to be critical to safe driving such as attention, executive functioning, processing speed, and motor coordination (Bishop et al. 2017; Corbett et al. 2009; Kenworthy et al. 2013; Lindsay 2016; Rosenthal et al. 2013; Yerys et al. 2013). Further, deficits in Theory of Mind—that is, the ability to recognize mental states (e.g., beliefs, emotions, knowledge) and understand that others have different perspectives and thoughts from oneself—may impede autistic drivers' ability to accurately perceive and predict how another road-user will behave (Sheppard et al. 2010). One study found that autistic individuals are less likely to identify social-hazards (e.g., a visible person) compared to non-social hazards (e.g., a car); however, other findings suggest this may be attributed to a difference in attentional processing while perceiving the hazard (Sheppard et al. 2010, 2016). Relatedly, during Theory of Mind tasks with eye tracking methods that require participants to interpret facial expressions, neurotypical individuals tend to focus on the mouth and eyes while autistic individuals tend to focus on the forehead or chin (Hopkins et al. 2011). Therefore, autistic individuals may not perceive fewer hazards, but instead have a harder time interpreting, processing, or prioritizing potential hazards if they include social factors (i.e., cyclists, pedestrians) (Monahan et al. 2013).

However, there are some features of autism that may make autistic drivers safer drivers than their typically developing peers. The inflexible rule-following behavior characteristic of many autistic individuals may make them less susceptible to intentional driving violations (i.e., speeding, running stop signs) (Chee et al. 2015). A recent study examined driving records of New Jersey residents and found that autistic drivers were 76% less likely to be at fault for a crash caused by speeding compared to non-autistic drivers (Curry et al. 2021). Autistic drivers also had a 32% lower rate of moving violations (i.e., speeding, following too closely) than non-autistic drivers. Recognizing the unique patterns of strengths and weakness in this population of drivers is essential in determining both how best to identify teens who will drive independently and the most effective driving training programs for those teens.

7.2.1 Who Are Autistic Drivers?

Almost 2 out of every 3 of teens on the autism spectrum are either interested in or currently driving based on parent-report (Huang et al. 2012). While driving can help autistic teens lead a more mobile and independent life, we know little about their driving experience. The first longitudinal study was recently conducted to determine the current rates and patterns of licensure among adolescents and young autistic individuals. The key findings have implications for parents, clinicians, driving educators, and researchers: 1 in 3 autistic adolescents received an intermediate license by age 21; the majority of autistic teens who receive a license do so in their 17th year, just like non-autistic teens; and the vast majority of autistic teens who do get a learner's permit go on to obtain a license to drive independently within two years (Curry et al. 2017). Since these teens who receive their learner's permit are getting licensed at nearly the same rate as typically developing teens, their families are committed to seeing the process through to independent driving.

Notably, there is a gap between autistic teens' *interest* in driving and the percentage of teens who are *actually* driving (Huang et al. 2012). This indicates a continued need for the research and support community to develop effective ways to ensure that autistic adolescents who want to obtain licensure are able to do so. There are certain factors that have been found to increase the likelihood of independent licensure among autistic adolescents interested in driving. These include placement in full time regular education, plans to attend college, a history of a paid job, and parents with experience teaching other teens to drive (Huang et al. 2012). In addition, the odds of licensure was eight times higher for autistic teens who included driving goals in their Individualized Education Plan (IEP) (Huang et al. 2012). Several key elements of an effective independent driving training plan have also been identified through interviews with specialized driving instructors (Myers et al. 2019).

Parents of autistic adolescents are critical in supporting both the decision-to-drive and the learning-to-drive process. In fact, professional specialized driving instructors view parents as integral partners in supporting their efforts to teach driving skills and promote independence. Parental involvement is important in both preparing teens for on-road instruction and supporting the development of specific driving skills (Myers et al. 2019). Parents should also support and prioritize their teen's independence before beginning the learning-to-drive process. Moreover, the driving instructors encourage parents to help their autistic adolescents develop life skills, such as mowing the lawn, cooking, and taking public transportation. These skills are critical in developing independence and making a successful transition to adulthood. Presently there are no standardized driving assessment approaches or instructional strategies to follow. This need for practicing driving skills may be particularly important for non-specialized instructors who are providing driving lessons to autistic teens without the benefit of additional training or access to specialized resources. However, driving instructors also recognize that specific driving education approaches will be tailored to meet the individual and unique needs of each autistic adolescent driver (Myers et al. 2019).

7.2.2 *The Decision to Drive*

For autistic individuals, the decision to pursue a driver's license is a milestone that other families might take for granted as a natural rite of passage for teenagers. When driving, there are no schedules to seek out, no waiting for buses in the rain or cold, and no need to pay for a cab or ride-sharing service. Driving is one of the most efficient ways to get around, particularly in non-urban settings. In some states, physicians and other professionals who diagnose and/or treat individuals with disabilities and medical disorders are required to report the names of patients ages 15 and older who have conditions that could impair their ability to safely operate a motor vehicle (Berger et al. 2000). Other states have different strategies for identifying and assessing drivers with impairments (e.g., self-monitoring and regulation of behavior). Parents and caregivers should talk to their network of support professionals, such as certified driving rehabilitation specialists—who are individuals who have specialized training in teaching autistic individuals to drive—when assessing specific skills associated with the decision to drive. The American Occupational Therapy Association also hosts an online database to help families locate a Driving Rehabilitation Specialist (visit www.aota.org for more information). Families should also consider that driving is much more than learning "the rules of the road" and being able to pass a licensing test. In actuality, it entails social judgment, motor coordination, planning, flexibility, the ability to focus, multi-tasking, prioritizing, anxiety management, and sensory sensitivity management.

Autism can affect social decision-making, information processing and attention to varying degrees. For example, consider the nonverbal communication that frequently occurs when multiple vehicles meet at a four-way stop sign. Drivers typically nod or motion to each other to communicate who is to go next since not everyone knows the rules related to order of entry into the intersection. Also, drivers must be aware that other drivers do not always act as expected. For example, a turn signal does not always mean the car is about to turn; it could mean the driver forgot to turn the signal off. Drivers must always be prepared for the unexpected, including rerouting (if a road is closed), checking in at speed limit or seat belt checkpoints, approaching emergency vehicles (with loud sirens and blinking lights), unsafe drivers, and breakdowns. All drivers must know how to respond if pulled over by the police, regardless of guilt or innocence. In addition, they must know what to do and who to call if the car breaks down or runs out of gas or if they are involved in an accident. Driving also requires being responsible for the maintenance of the car, such as making sure the car is filled with sufficient gas in the tank, the tires are properly inflated, and all parts (for example, turn signals) are functioning appropriately. Perhaps even more important are the strategic level decisions required for safe driving—deciding if it is safe to drive in bad weather, determining if you are in a fit state to drive physically or emotionally. These skills require forethought and goal-directed behavior and should be carefully assessed and developed before autistic individuals begin driving independently.

7.2.3 Challenges and Barriers to Driving

Parents are appropriately concerned, as autistic teens may have characteristics that place them at risk for unsafe driving behaviors, like getting lost in the details of the road, difficulty recognizing the cues of others on the road, or inattention (Chee et al. 2015). Current research examining the actual driving performance of autistic teens is mixed but several areas of concern are consistently mentioned: anxiety, processing speed, and social skill (Lindsay 2016; Wilson et al. 2018).

Anxiety is one of the most commonly reported driving barriers for autistic individuals (Almberg et al. 2015; Cox et al. 2012). Anxiety disorder presents as a disproportionate fear or adverse reaction to relatively nonthreatening environmental stimuli and is a common co-occurring condition seen in autistic individuals (National Institute of Mental Health [NIMH] 2016; White et al. 2009). Although prevalence rates of anxiety disorders in the autistic population have been varied, ranging from 47% to 84% (Gillot et al. 2001; White et al. 2009), several studies have found higher rates of clinical and subclinical levels of anxiety in autistic individuals as compared to typically developing groups (Bellini 2004; Gillot et al. 2001; Vohra et al. 2016). Within the population of autistic individuals, it has also been found that those without intellectual disability exhibit particularly high levels of anxiety (Bellini 2004; Gillot et al. 2001). This is an especially pertinent issue as they are the subgroup of autistic individuals who are mostly likely to drive independently and heightened anxiety may keep them from getting a driving license (Chee et al. 2015; Curry et al. 2017; Lindsay 2016).

There is a large body of literature suggesting that anxiety has a negative impact on general task performance (Hembree 1988; Holdnack et al. 2011; Seipp 2007). Several theories have been proposed to explain this relationship (Taylor et al. 2008). One of the most popular of these theories is the Processing Efficiency Theory (PET), which posits that the worry and constant monitoring of potentially harmful stimuli reduce the efficiency of working memory, processing speed and subsequently task performance (Eysenck and Calvo 1992). Several of the cognitive domains impacted by high levels of anxiety are critical to the task of driving including working memory and information processing (Beck and Clark 1997; Eysenck and Calvo 1992; Pacheco-Unguetti et al. 2010). Higher levels of anxiety may increase driving errors (i.e., failures of observation), lapses (i.e., absent-minded behaviors), violations (i.e., deliberate departures from safe driving behaviors) and aggressive violations (Shahar 2009). Anxiety has also been associated with more self-reported driving errors and poorer simulated driving performance (e.g., poor steering control) (Matthews et al. 1991, 1998). However, it has also been suggested that some anxiety may actually improve task performance by increasing awareness and alertness (Taylor et al. 2008).

Another highly important skill for safe driving is visual processing speed, which is defined as "the amount of time needed to make a correct judgment about a visual stimulus" (i.e., detecting a target, identifying a target's spatial location) (Owsley 2013). As this ability is used constantly during the task of driving (e.g., detecting hazards in the environment, judging the spatial positions of other vehicles), visual processing speed is a key skill for navigating the driving environment safely (Anstey et al. 2012). Typically developing, experienced drivers are better able to quickly identify important, safety-relevant aspects of the driving environment (e.g., the cars in front of them, pedestrian crosswalks, traffic lights and road signs) compared to novice drivers (Almberg et al. 2015; Borowsky et al. 2010).

Experienced drivers' increased attention to important areas of the driving environment and their ability to quickly scan the scene for hazards provides them with adequate information to drive safely and allows them to react more quickly to avoid these hazardous situations (Almberg et al. 2015; Borowsky et al. 2010). This motor visual processing speed has been shown in previous research to be underdeveloped in autistic individuals (Corbett et al. 2009; Kenworthy et al. 2013; Oliveras-Rentas et al. 2012; Yi et al. 2012). In the real-world driving environment, the inability to rapidly process a large amount of visual information in an environment and identify important target items (e.g., traffic lights, other cars, pedestrians, stop signs, etc.) can result in an increased risk of motor vehicle collision. The combination of processing speed impairments already present in autistic individuals along with the reduced efficiency of information processing caused by anxiety may make the task of driving especially difficult for this population. Especially in the context of driving, these deficiencies may also be compounded by the effect of social difficulties.

Although each individual is in their own vehicle, the network of drivers on the roadway is an undeniably social environment (Benson et al. 2010; Kulp and Sortor 2003). The existence of this vast social ecosystem is contingent on the successful interactions of hundreds of drivers running smoothly. This ecosystem includes not only drivers, but also other road users, including cyclists and pedestrians. The often sudden and sometimes subtle exchanges between drivers and other road users can be the difference between a life or death outcome. This complex social exchange between pedestrians and drivers can occur in something as indirect as a pedestrian smiling at a driver. Surprisingly, research has shown that drivers were more likely to stop for and drove more slowly approaching a pedestrian who was smiling compared to one who was not (Guéguena et al. 2016). This suggests that non-verbal communication—even something as subtle as a smile indicating acknowledgement of one's presence—can alter the relationship between road users. The use of body language as a form of non-verbal communication is automatic in drivers, but may not be in autistic drivers. Numerous studies have revealed significant impairments in the interpretation of body language as a form of communication for autistic individuals compared to typically developing individuals (Centelles et al. 2013; Klin et al. 2003; Zalla et al. 2013). These deficits are less apparent when autistic participants are specifically asked to identify the meaning of body cues in a laboratory setting, compared to when placed in naturalistic settings when the impairments become much more distinct (Zalla et al. 2013). The interpretation of body language comes into play for drivers most when encountering other road users (e.g., pedestrians or cyclists). Interpreting and anticipating the actions of pedestrians and cyclists is an essential skill for drivers to possess to maintain safety. Without the ability to anticipate and interpret the actions of other drivers, getting around in the environment, especially the driving environment, may be exceedingly more challenging for autistic drivers.

7.2.4 The Learning-to-Drive Process

Due to the complex nature of autism and the vast diversity of presentation from person to person, the learning-to-drive process for autistic teens and young adults can be challenging. Although each autistic driver's needs are unique, researchers have begun to characterize the learner period through parent and driving instructors' perspectives. The majority (70%) of parents with autistic teens who were driving or trying to receive their driver's license, reported that their child's autism "moderately" to "extremely" negatively impacted their child's driving abilities (Cox et al. 2012). These same parents identified the ability to multitask (e.g., merging while maintaining speed), awareness of traffic, use of mirrors and the ability to maintain lane position as the most difficult (rated as "very difficult') skills to teach their autistic child (Cox et al. 2012). Turning, controlling speed, and braking were also rated as "difficult" tasks when teaching their child to drive. Parents also rated the impact of seven characteristics commonly associated with autism on their adolescent's driving abilities, and reported that "non-verbal communication" and "unexpected changes in routine" were the most problematic for driving (Cox et al. 2012). Adjusting to unfamiliar situations is also one of the most commonly reported problematic skills (Almberg et al. 2015). Qualitative data from this study echo many of the concerns that parents of autistic teens have expressed in previous research. Many of these concerns were also voiced when asking autistic teens directly about their driving training. For example, one teen said, "You have to learn to think, to anticipate that a child may run out on the road from behind a hedge or so... yeah, it's hard. I sort of think I'm in control but my instructor anticipates many more hazards than I do, and brakes before I understand why" (Almberg et al. 2015). Autistic teens also self-reported "interacting with other drivers" and "interpreting traffic situations" as some of the most difficult driving skills (Almberg et al. 2015). When these same teens' driving instructors were questioned about the driving situations that were most challenging for autistic drivers, they cited the inflexibility and rule following characteristics of ASD as major barriers to driving. The ability to drive is vital for success in achieving the independent lifestyle desired by the majority of autistic individuals and with proper targeted programming, many of these barriers to driving can be overcome (Gaylord et al. 2005).

Commentary driving is an effective, safe and empirically supported method of driver training that may prove especially useful for autistic individuals (Myers et al. 2019). Commentary driving involves the parent or caregiver narrating what is happening as they drive with their autistic teen sitting in the car as a passenger. Then, the autistic teen takes over and narrates driving instructions to the person driving, following the model of their parent or caregiver. This allows the autistic individual to safely learn how to scan the driving environment and plan driving maneuvers ahead of time. This technique also allows driving instructors and parents to safely gauge the skill level of their teen and focus on skills that need improvement.

Although the learning-to-drive process can be daunting for parents of autistic teens, there are resources available to families. Most states in the U.S. have state-level driver training programs for autistic individuals through Vocational Rehabilitation Services, which may provide financial support for specialized instruction (Monahan et al. 2013). These programs provide a comprehensive evaluation of skills and allow autistic drivers to work with an instructor one-on-one to ensure adequate time to successfully learn safe driving skills. Certified Driver Rehabilitation Specialists or Occupational Therapists (OTs) can also provide specialized training and safe driving advice for adolescent autistic drivers. Families of autistic teens should work with their autism support network and general physician to discover what vocational rehabilitation driving assistance services are available in their area.

7.2.5 Police Interactions

For autistic individuals, difficulties with social interactions may make communicating with strangers a challenging experience. When the stranger is a police officer, the encounter can quickly become dangerous for everyone involved. Unfortunately, there have been a number of serious incidents between autistic individuals and police officers. For example, in Florida in 2016, police shot a group home therapist in the leg while answering a 911 call about a man who was believed to be mentally ill and armed. In reality, the therapist was trying to help a severely autistic man. Police shot at the man, whose "weapon" turned out to be a toy truck, resulting in the bullet hitting and wounding the therapist (Rabin 2016). In another event that occurred in 2016, an autistic man failed to obey a police officer's commands after being pulled over and then drove away. After being stopped again, he got out of the car, again failed to obey the police and was fatally shot (Schwien and Downing 2016). These devastating incidents illustrate a growing concern among individuals and families in the autism community, as well as law enforcement and behavioral health professionals. Some of the core symptoms of autism spectrum disorder—social anxiety, unusual gestures, reduced eye contact and difficulty processing verbal and body language—can resemble a police officer's standard profile of a suspicious person. Add flashing lights and the blare of a siren, and the environment can be paralyzing for someone with autism, who may have extreme sensitivity to light, sound or touch. Research shows that 1 in 5 young autistic individuals will be stopped and questioned by police before age 21 (Rava et al. 2017). Therefore, teaching autistic individuals at an early age how to safely interact with police is critical. While many police departments around the country offer training to help officers recognize and respond to people who have social and cognitive challenges, these trainings are often not mandated, and autistic individuals rarely receive training that involves active participation (Love et al. 2020).

7.2.6 Recommendations for Families and Clinicians

Although further research is needed to understand how families make the decision for autistic individuals to drive and how clinicians and driving educators can best provide support, a few recommendations can ease the transition to independent transportation, providing autistic individuals the highest probability of success.

(1) Parents should initiate the conversation about driving with their child early. A healthcare provider can help to guide that conversation with questions regarding readiness to drive. During this visit, parents should address any concerns, such as attention or sensory issues.
(2) Parents may want to consider seeking the advice of a certified driver rehabilitation specialist who has training in working with individuals with special needs or an occupational therapist who is a driving specialist.
(3) If the autistic teen has symptoms of ADHD, parents should consider medication options with their teen's healthcare provider.
(4) When beginning parent-supervised practice driving, parents should log at the minimum the amount of practice driving hours required by their state while ideally aiming to exceed that number. Parents should also use evidence-based programs, such as the TeenDrivingPlan Practice Guide, created by the Teen Driver Safety Research team at Children's Hospital of Philadelphia (Mirman et al. 2014) or driver training applications for smartphones (e.g., AutoCoach 2.0[2] or DriveFocus[3]).
(5) Healthcare providers should encourage families to add driving-related goals to their teen's Individualized Education Plan one to two years before the permit stage and while seeking extra support from the school.

Other crucial information needed to inform programs to help teach autistic teens lead a more mobile life include: the extent to which autistic adolescents get licensed and how their driving outcomes compare to neurotypical adolescents; whether families feel informed and supported while making driving decisions; how families and the adolescent are or will be affected by not driving; and the extent to which healthcare providers or driver educators are involved in the process.

In addition, driving simulators may also serve as an excellent tool for reducing driving anxiety, especially since they allow individuals to experience and interact with risky, anxiety-provoking driving situations in a safe and ethical way. Not only has previous research demonstrated the usefulness of virtual reality (VR) in reducing anxiety symptoms, but also VR driving environments have shown promise in training and improving driving performance in novice autistic drivers (Bian et al. 2013; Cox et al. 2017). Autistic individuals may also benefit greatly from the implementation of proven, therapeutic techniques to specifically target driving anxiety, such as cognitive behavior therapy (CBT) (Bruggink et al. 2016).

---

[2] https://www.shepherd.org/about/injuryprevention/autocoach.

[3] https://drivefocus.com/.

Professionals in the autism field are also turning to VR to offer individuals the opportunity to practice safe interactions with a police officer in simulations that are similar to real-life experiences (McCleery et al. 2020). The goal of this work is to develop behavioral support and materials to help autistic individuals practice interacting with police officers across a variety of different contexts—tall police officers, short police officers, day, night, urban, suburban. An important part of the training will be learning what to do and what not to do, while also having the opportunity to practice the right behaviors. One study established safety of the VR platform for teaching police interaction skills to autistic individuals and demonstrated feasibility with high user engagement and enjoyment, as well as found the equipment easy to navigate (McCleery et al. 2020). This study sets the stage for future pilot studies to demonstrate the intervention's efficacy.

7.3 Other Forms of Transportation

Given the importance of transportation for increased access to community activities, education, health care, employment, and social relationships, it is critical that we meet the transportation needs of autistic individuals who are uninterested or unable to drive independently. Survey data suggest that the majority of autistic individuals rely on parents or caregivers as their primary source of transportation (Feeley 2010). As a result, it is difficult for these individuals to travel, but it also increases the time and economic burden, as well as the employment and social opportunities for their families. Although public transit (i.e., trains, subways and bus systems) is a commonly used form of transportation for the general public in urban areas, it is often unavailable or not feasible in rural areas of the country. Currently, the autistic community is underserved by public transportation in many areas of the country due to the complexities of navigating it or lack of accessibility (Rezae et al. 2019). Autistic individuals are not always well trained to use public transit and may have difficulty understanding how to use the systems. Further, other transportation options such as walking or biking are dangerous in these rural regions. Because of these challenges, many autistic individuals are unable to get to and from work, school, health care or recreational activities or errands, which can lead to a decreased quality of life. In urban areas, public transportation accessibility is better for autistic individuals, but still offers a level of confusion and anxiety because it is often difficult to navigate. In the autism population, barriers to using public transportation include difficulty with or lack of speech; social interaction difficulties; sensory sensitivities; severe repetitive behaviors or needs for sameness; and coexisting medical or mental health issues (Feeley 2010). Further, some of the most prevalent concerns for families of autistic adolescents in using public transportation is safety in traveling alone and awareness of location and knowing when to get off and on to arrive at their destination (Rezae et al. 2019).

Ride sharing programs, such as Lyft and Uber offer a new mode of independent mobility option for the autism population. These programs provide several notable advantages over public transit: (1) the ability to pre-plan routes removes the confusion that comes with determining when to get on and off transit systems; (2) destination pick-up and drop-off eliminates the need to navigate to train or bus stations; and (3) the cash-free payment system provides a level of safety absent in some taxi systems. Although ride sharing does provide a solution for occasional travel, the cost of using them may not be feasible for daily travel. Little research has been conducted in this relatively new area of transportation, especially as it relates to the potential benefits to autistic individuals.

7.3.1 Addressing Challenges of Other Transportation

Travel training can help autistic teens learn to use public transportation and know what to do when unexpected events occur. The Individuals with Disabilities Education Act (IDEA) and its regulations include travel training in the definition of special education (U.S. Department of Education 2017). Travel training is instruction that enables teens with disabilities to develop an awareness of the environment in which they live and to learn the skills necessary to move effectively and safely from one place to another within that environment. Travel training is often included in the transition plan of a student's IEP, as it is a necessary component for preparing a student for employment and independent living in the community. Travel training usually consists of both classroom-based and community-based instruction. During the training, an autistic student will learn how to use maps and schedules for trip planning, which are often available as a paper brochure and online (perhaps even in a smart phone app that can alert the user to when trains are running late or are canceled). The student will also learn how to purchase tickets, including both exchanging payment and communicating with transportation employees. Safety precautions will be taught (for example, how to cross streets, how to recognize and respond to danger, how to recognize the need for assistance and request help from an appropriate source), and scenarios, such as delayed trains, trains that do not make anticipated stops, going the wrong way, and getting off at the wrong stop, will be role-played. In the community, students practice the skills, accompanied by a travel instructor, who will lessen support as the student progresses.

In Philadelphia, a peer-to-peer training program shows promise in teaching autistic young adults to navigate the SEPTA public train lines. The program connects those on the autism spectrum to mentors participating in the program to increase education about public transportation safety and usage. Autistic individuals first learn about street safety, signs and basic travel fundamentals. Then they are paired with a mentor for 10–12 one-on-one sessions that consist of traveling on public transportation. The pilot program partners with SEPTA to waive rider fees to help mitigate the financial costs associated with real-world public transit training (Brown 2019).

Technological solutions are also being developed and tested to address some of the concerns of autistic individuals and their families. Smartphone applications provide a unique opportunity for widespread implementation of assistive systems to navigating public transit. These applications allow autistic individuals to plan their trips ahead of time with or without the assistance of parents or caregivers and use the application as a guide during travel (Rezae et al. 2019). Virtual reality games have also shown promise in increasing autistic individuals' knowledge about the process of riding a bus and reducing anxiety about travel (Simões et al. 2018).

References

Almberg, M., H. Selander, M. Falkmer, S. Vaz, M. Ciccarelli, and T. Falkmer. 2015. Experiences of facilitators or barriers in driving education from learner and novice drivers with ADHD or ASD and their driving instructors. *Developmental Neurorehabilitation* 20 (2): 59–67. https://doi.org/10.3109/17518423.2015.1058299.

Anstey, K.J., M.S. Horswell, J.M. Wood, and C. Hatherly. 2012. The role of cognitive and visual abilities as predictors in the multifactorial model of driving safety. *Accident: Analysis and Prevention* 45: 766–774.

Beck, A.T., and D.A. Clark. 1997. An information processing model of anxiety: Automatic and strategic processes. *Behavior Research and Therapy* 35 (1): 49–58. https://doi.org/10.1016/S0005-7967(96)00069-1.

Bellini, S. 2004. Social skill deficits and anxiety in high-functioning adolescents with autism spectrum disorders. *Focus on Autism and Other Developmental Disabilities* 19 (2): 78–86.

Benson N., D.M. Hulac, and J.H. Kranzler. 2010. Independent examination of the Wechsler adult intelligence scale—fourth edition (WAIS-IV): What does the WAIS-IV measure? *Psychological Assessment* 22 (1): 121–130. https://doi.org/10.1037/a0017767.

Berger, J.T., F. Rosner, P. Kark, and A.J. Bennett. 2000. Reporting by physicians of impaired drivers and potentially impaired drivers. *Journal of General Internal Medicine* 15 (9): 667–672. https://doi.org/10.1046/j.1525-1497.2000.04309.x.

Bian, D., J.W. Wade, et al. 2013. A novel virtual reality driving environment for autism intervention. Paper presented at the International Conference on Universal Access in Human-Computer Interaction, Las Vegas, Nevada, 21–26 July 2013.

Bishop, H.J., F.J. Biasini, and D. Stavrinos. 2017. Social and non-social hazard response in drivers with autism spectrum disorder. *Journal of Autism and Developmental Disorders* 47 (4): 905–917. https://doi.org/10.1007/s10803-016-2992-1.

Borowsky, A., D. Shinar, and T. Oron-Gilad. 2010. Age, skill, and hazard perception in driving. *Accident Analysis & Prevention* 42 (4): 1240–1249. https://doi.org/10.1016/j.aap.2010.02.001.

Brown, T. 2019. New program teaches commuters with ASD public transportation. *Temple News*. https://temple-news.com/new-program-teaches-commuters-with-asd-public-transportation/. Accessed 22 Feb 2021.

Bruggink, A., S. Huisman, R. Vuijk, V. Kraaij, and N. Garnefski. 2016. Cognitive emotion regulation, anxiety and depression in adults with autism spectrum disorder. *Research in Autism Spectrum Disorders* 22: 34–44. https://doi.org/10.1016/j.rasd.2015.11.003.

Centelles, L., C. Assaiante, K. Etchegoyhen, M. Bouvard, and C. Schmitz. 2013. From action to interaction: Exploring the contribution of body motion cues to social understanding in typical development and in autism spectrum disorders. *Journal of Autism and Developmental Disorders* 43 (5): 1140–1150. https://doi.org/10.1007/s10803-012-1655-0.

Center for Disease Control and Prevention. 2018. Autism Spectrum Disorder (ASD): Facts about ASD. http://www.cdc.gov/ncbddd/autism/data.html Accessed 22 Feb 2021.

Chee, D.Y., H.C. Lee, M. Falkmer, T. Barnett, O. Falkmer, J. Siljehav, and T. Falkmer. 2015. Viewpoints on driving of individuals with and without autism spectrum disorder. *Developmental Neurorehabilitation* 18 (1): 26–36. https://doi.org/10.3109/17518423.2014.964377.

Corbett, B.A., L.J. Constantine, R. Hendren, D. Rocke, and S. Ozonoff. 2009. Examining executive functioning in children with autism spectrum disorder, attention deficit hyperactivity disorder and typical development. *Psychiatry Research* 166 (23): 210–222.

Cox, D.J., T. Brown, V. Ross, M. Moncrief, R. Schmitt, G. Gaffney, and R. Reeve. 2017. Can youth with autism spectrum disorder use virtual reality driving simulation training to evaluate and improve driving performance? An exploratory study. *Journal of Autism and Developmental Disorders* 47 (8): 2544–2555. https://doi.org/10.1007/s10803-015-2677-1.

Cox, N.B., R.E. Reeve, S.M. Cox, and D.J. Cox. 2012. Brief report: Driving and young adults with ASD: Parents' experiences. *Journal of Autism and Developmental Disorders* 42 (10): 2257–2262.

Curry, A.E., K.B. Metzger, M.E. Carey, E.B. Sartin, P. Huang, and B.E. Yerys. 2021. Motor vehicle crashes and traffic violations among autistic adolescent and young adult drivers. *Digital Journal of the American Academy of Child and Adolescent Psychiatry*. https://doi.org/10.1016/j.jaac.2021.01.001.

Curry, A.E., B.E. Yerys, P. Huang, and K.B. Metzger. 2017. Longitudinal study of driver licensing rates among adolescents and young adults with autism spectrum disorder. *Autism* 22 (4): 479–488. https://doi.org/10.1177/1362361317699586.

Danziger, L. 1999. A dynamic economy with costly price adjustments. *American Economy Review* 89 (4): 878–901. https://doi.org/10.1257/aer.89.4.878.

Dickerson, A.E., L.J. Molnar, D.W. Eby, G. Adler, M. Bédard, M. Berg-Weger, et al. 2007. Transportation and aging: A research agenda for advancing safe mobility. *The Gerontologist* 47 (5): 578–590. https://doi.org/10.1093/geront/47.5.578.

Eysenck, M.W., and M.G. Calvo. 1992. Anxiety and performance: The processing efficiency theory. *Cognition and Emotion* 6: 409–434.

Feeley, C. (2010). Evaluating the transportation needs and accessibility issues for adults on the autism spectrum in New Jersey. Paper presented at the Transportation Research Board 89th Annual Meeting, Washington, DC, 10–14 January 2010.

Gaylord, V., A. Abeson, E. Bosk, J. Timmons, and S. Lazarus. 2005. Meeting transportation needs of youth and adults with developmental disabilities. *Impact* 18 (3): 1–34.

Geller, L.L., and M. Greenberg. 2009. Managing the transition process from high school to college and beyond: Challenges for individuals, families, and society. *Social Work in Mental Health* 8: 92–116. https://doi.org/10.1080/15332980902932466.

Gillot, A., F. Furniss, and A. Walter. 2001. Anxiety in high-functioning children with autism. *Autism* 5 (3): 277–286.

Guéguena, N., C. Eyssartierb, and S. Meineria. 2016. A pedestrian's smile and drivers' behavior: When a smile increases careful driving. *Journal of Safety Research* 56: 83–88. https://doi.org/10.1016/j.jsr.2015.12.005.

Hembree, R. 1988. Correlates, causes, effects and treatment of test anxiety. *Review of Educational Research* 58 (1): 47–77. https://doi.org/10.3102/00346543058001047.

Holdnack, J.A., X. Zhou, G.J. Larrabee, S.R. Millis, and T.A. Salthouse. 2011. Confirmatory factor analysis of the WASI-IV/WMS-IV. *Assessment* 18 (2): 178–191. https://doi.org/10.1177/1073191110393106.

Hopkins, I.M., M.W. Gower, T.A. Perez, D.S. Smith, F.R. Amthor, F.C. Wimsatt, and F.J. Biasini. 2011. Avatar assistant: Improving social skills in students with an ASD through a computer-based intervention. *Journal of Autism and Developmental Disorders* 41: 1543–1555.

Huang, P., T. Kao, A.E. Curry, and D.R. Durbin. 2012. Factors associated with driving in teens with autism spectrum disorders. *Journal of Developmental & Behavioral Pediatrics* 33 (1): 70–74.

Interagency Autism Coordinating Committee. 2017. 2017 Strategic plan for autism spectrum disorders. Department of Health and Human Services Interagency Autism Coordinating Committee. http://iacc.hhs.gov/strategic-plan/2011/index.shtml.

Kenworthy, L., B.E. Yerys, R. Weinblatt, D.N. Abrams, and G. L. Wallace. 2013. Motor demands impact speed of information processing in autism spectrum disorders. *Neuropsychology* 27 (5): 529–536. https://doi.org/10.1037/a0033599.

Klin, A., W. Jones, R. Schultz, and F. Volkmar. 2003. The enactive mind, or from actions to cognition: Lessons from autism. *Philosophical Transactions of the Royal Society of London. Series B: Biological Sciences* 358 (1430): 345–360.

Kulp, M.T., and J.M. Sortor. 2003. Clinical value of the Beery visual-motor integration supplemental tests of visual perception and motor coordination. *Optometry and Vision Science* 80 (4): 312–315. 1040-5488/03/8004-0312/0.

Lindsay, S. 2016. Systematic review of factors affecting driving and motor vehicle transportation among people with autism spectrum disorder. *Disability and Rehabilitation* 39 (9): 837–846. https://doi.org/10.3109/09638288.2016.1161849.

Love, A.M.A., E.L. Usher, M.D. Toland, K.S. Railey, J.M. Campbell, and A.D. Spriggs. 2020. Measuring police officer self-efficacy for working with individuals with autism spectrum disorder. *Journal of Autism and Developmental Disorders*. https://doi.org/10.1007/s10803-020-04613-1.

Lubin, A. (2012). Persons with disabilities seeking employment and public transportation: Findings of a New Jersey survey. Disability and Work. http://www.heldrich.rutgers.edu/sites/default/files/products/uploads/Public_Transportation_Disabilities_Survey_Brief_0.pdf. Accessed 22 Feb 2021.

Lucas, K., and G. Currie. 2012. Developing socially inclusive transportation policy: Transferring the United Kingdom policy approach to the State of Victoria? *Transportation* 39 (1): 151–173.

Matthews, G., L. Dorn, and A.I. Glendon. 1991. Personality correlates of driver stress. *Personality and Individual Differences* 12 (6): 535–549. https://doi.org/10.1016/0191-8869(91)90248-A.

Matthews, G., L. Dorn, T.W. Hoyes, D.R. Davies, A.I. Glendon, and R.G. Taylor. 1998. Driving stress and performance on a driving simulator. *Journal of Human Factors and Ergonomics Society* 40 (1): 136–149. https://doi.org/10.1518/001872098779480569.

McCleery, J., A. Zitter, R. Solorzano, S. Turnaciolgu, J. Miller, V. Ravindran, and J. Parish-Morris. 2020. Safety and feasibility of an immersive virtual reality intervention program for teaching police interactions skills to adolescents and adults with autism. *Autism Research* 13 (1): 1418–1424.

Mirman, J.H., D.W. Albert, A.E. Curry, F.K. Winston, M.C.F. Thiel, and D.R. Durbin. 2014. TeenDrivingPlan effectiveness: The effect of quantity and diversity of supervised practice on teens' driving performance. *Journal of Adolescent Health* 55 (5): 620–626. https://doi.org/10.1016/j.jadohealth.2014.04.010.

Monahan, M., S. Classen, and P.V. Helsel. 2013. Pre-driving evaluation of a teen with attention deficit hyperactivity disorder and autism spectrum disorder. *Canadian Journal of Occupational Therapy* 80 (1): 35–41. https://doi.org/10.1177/0008417412474221.

Myers, R.K., J.M. Bonsu, M.E. Carey, B.E. Yerys, C.J. Mollen, and A.E. Curry. 2019. Teaching autistic adolescents and young adults to drive: Perspectives of specialized driving instructors. *Autism in Adulthood* 1 (3): 202–209. https://doi.org/10.1089/aut.2018.0054.

National Institute of Mental Health [NIMH]. 2016. Anxiety disorders. https://www.nimh.nih.gov/health/topics/anxiety-disorders/index.shtml.

Oliveras-Rentas, R.E., L. Kenworthy, R.B. Roberson 3rd, A. Martin, and G.L. Wallace (2012) WISC-IV profile in high-functioning autism spectrum disorders: Impaired processing speed is associated with increased autism communication symptoms and decreased adaptive communication abilities. *Journal of Autism and Developmental Disorders* 42 (5): 655–664. https://doi.org/10.1007/s10803-011-1289-7.

Owsley, C. 2013. Visual processing speed. *Vision Research* 90: 52–56. https://doi.org/10.1016/j.visres.2012.11.014.

Pacheco-Unguetti, A., A. Acosta, A. Callejas, and J. Lupianez. 2010. Attention and anxiety: Different attentional functioning under state and trait anxiety. *Psychological Science* 21 (2): 298–304. https://doi.org/10.1177/0956797609359624.

Rabin, C. 2016. Charles Kinsey was shot less than six minutes after police arrived. *Miami Herald*. https://www.miamiherald.com/news/local/crime/article94009242.html. Accessed 22 Feb 2021.

Rava, J.A., P. Shattuck, J. Rast, and A. Roux. 2017. The prevalence and correlates of involvement in the criminal justice system among youth on the autism spectrum. *Journal of Autism and Developmental Disorders* 47 (2): 340–346. https://doi.org/10.1007/s10803-016-2958-3.

Rezae, M., McMeekin, D., Tan, T., Krishna, A., Lee, H., & Falkmer, T. (2019). Public transport planning tool for users on the autism spectrum: From concept to prototype. *Digital Disability and Rehabilitation: Assistive Technology*. https://doi.org/10.1080/17483107.2019.1646818.

Rosenthal, M., G.L. Wallace, R. Lawson, M.C. Wills, E. Dixon, B.E. Yerys, and L. Kenworthy. 2013. Impairments in real world executive function increases from childhood to adolescence in autism spectrum disorder. *Neuropsychology* 27 (1): 13–18. https://doi.org/10.1037/a0031299.

Roux, A.M., P.T. Shattuck, J.E. Rast, J.A. Rava, and K.A Anderson. (2015). National autism indicators report: Transition into young adulthood. *A J Drexel Autism Institute*. https://drexel.edu/autismoutcomes/publications-and-reports/publications/National-Autism-Indicators-Report-Transition-to-Adulthood/. Accessed 22 Feb 2021.

Schwien, N., and S. Downing. 2016. Man's death 'tragic, inconceivable'. *Hays Daily News*. https://www.hdnews.net/article/20160820/news/308209802. Accessed 22 Feb 2021.

Seipp, B. 2007. Anxiety and academic performance: A meta-analysis of findings. *Anxiety Research* 4 (1): 27–41. https://doi.org/10.1080/08917779108248762.

Shahar, A. 2009. Self-reported driving behaviors as a function of trait anxiety. *Accident Analysis & Prevention* 41 (2): 241–245. https://doi.org/10.1016/j.aap.2008.11.004.

Sheppard, E., D. Ropar, G. Underwood, and E. Van Loon. 2010. Brief report: Driving hazard perception in autism. *Journal of Autism and Developmental Disorders* 40 (4): 504–508.

Sheppard, E., E. van Loon, G. Underwood, and D. Ropar. 2016. Attentional differences in a driving hazard perception task in adults with autism spectrum disorder. *Journal of Autism and Developmental Disorders* 47 (2): 405–414. https://doi.org/10.1007/s10803-016-2965-4.

Simões, M., M. Bernardes, F. Barros, and M. Castelo-Branco. 2018. Virtual travel training for autism spectrum disorder: Proof-of-concept interventional study. *JMIR Serious Games* 6 (1): e5. https://doi.org/10.2196/games.8428.

Syed, S.T., B.S. Gerber, and L.K. Sharp. 2013. Traveling towards disease: Transportation barriers to health care access. *Journal of Community Health* 38 (5): 976–993. https://doi.org/10.1007/s10900-013-9681-1.

Taylor, J.E., F.P. Deane, and J. Podd. 2008. The relationship between driving anxiety and driving skill: A review of human factors and anxiety-performance theories to clarify future research needs. *New Zealand Journal of Psychology* 37 (1): 28–37.

Taylor, L.T., and N.A. Henninger. 2015. Frequency and correlates of service access among youth with autism transitioning to adulthood. *Journal of Autism and Developmental Disorders* 45 (1): 179–191. https://doi.org/10.1007/s10803-014-2203-x.

U.S. Department of Education. 2017. Sec. 300.39 Special education. https://sites.ed.gov/idea/regs/b/a/300.39. Accessed 22 Feb 2021.

Vohra, R., S. Madhavan, and U. Sambamoorthi. 2016. Comorbidity prevalence, healthcare utilization, and expenditures of Medicaid enrolled adults with autism spectrum disorders. *Autism* 21 (8): 995–1009. https://doi.org/10.1177/1362361316665222.

Wallace, R., P. Hughes-Cromwick, H. Mull, and S. Khasnabis. 2005. Access to health care and nonemergency medical transportation: Two missing links. *Transportation Research Record: Journal of the Transportation Research Board* 1924: 76–84. https://doi.org/10.1177/0361198105192400110.

White, S.W., D. Oswald, T. Ollendick, and L. Scahill. 2009. Anxiety in children and adolescents with autism spectrum disorders. *Clinical Psychology Review* 29 (3): 216–229. https://doi.org/10.1016/j.cpr.2009.01.003.

Wilson, N.J., H.C. Lee, S. Vaz, P. Vindin, and R. Cordier. 2018. Scoping review of the driving behaviour of and driver training programs for people on the autism spectrum. *Behavioural Neurology* 2018: 1–17. https://doi.org/10.1155/2018/6842306.

Winston, F.K., and T. Senerrick. 2006. Competent independent driving as an archetypal task of adolescence. *Injury Prevention* 12: 1–3. https://doi.org/10.1136/ip.2006.012765.

Yerys, B.E., L. Kenworthy, K.F. Jankowski, J. Strang, and G.L. Wallace. 2013. Separate components of emotional go/no-go performance relate to autism versus attention symptoms in children with autism. *Neuropsychology* 27 (5): 537–545. https://doi.org/10.1037/a0033615.

Yi, L., Y. Liu, Y. Li, Y. Fan, D. Huang, and D. Gao. 2012. Visual scanning patterns during the dimensional change card sorting task in children with autism spectrum disorder. *Autism Research and Treatment* 2012: 1–11. https://doi.org/10.1155/2012/123053.

Zalla, T., N. Labruyere, and N. Georgieff. 2013. Perceiving goals and actions in individuals with autism spectrum disorders. *Journal of Autism and Developmental Disorders* 43 (10): 2353–2365.

Chapter 8
Autism and Voting Rights

Eugene Schnitzler and Elizabeth M. Yang

Abstract Voting rights are viewed as sacrosanct in the U.S. Unless one is incarcerated or is deemed incompetent, one possesses the right to vote. An examination of voting rights for autistic adults is best seen through the lens of the history of voting rights in the U.S. as juxtaposed with the slow and turbulent movement for greater inclusion of disadvantaged and marginalized groups in society. One must consider what characteristics of an autistic individual serve to create a state of disenfranchisement. Why are some autistic individuals denied the right to vote? The answer lies in a determination of mental incapacity, whether or not an individual is unable to make their own decisions due to illness or disability. Our laws should be drafted in a manner that seeks inclusion of as many eligible voters, as opposed to exclusion.

The right to vote for autistic citizens has only recently been considered as a credible concept worthy of debate. Historically, the developmentally disabled have been excluded from day-to-day life by institutionalization, segregation, incarceration and even eugenic sterilization. Regulations disenfranchising the "insane," "idiots," and "mentally incapacitated" (terms now viewed as offensive) were incorporated into most state constitutions and reiterated by numerous state and local statutes (Shiner and Ochs 2000). An examination of voting rights for autistic adults is best seen through the lens of the history of voting rights in the U.S. as juxtaposed with the slow and turbulent movement for greater inclusion of disadvantaged and marginalized groups in society.

E. Schnitzler (✉)
Loyola University Medical Center, Maywood, IL, USA
e-mail: eschnitzler@lumc.edu

E. M. Yang
WStrong, LLC, Reston, VA, USA

N. Elster and K. Parsi (eds.), *Transitioning to Adulthood with Autism: Ethical, Legal and Social Issues*, The International Library of Bioethics 91,
https://doi.org/10.1007/978-3-030-91487-5_8

8.1 Historical Perspective: Disability Rights and Voting Rights

Following the examples of the Civil Rights and Women's Liberation Movements of the 1960s, the Disability Rights Movement began in the 1970s and has been evolving ever since. The Americans with Disabilities Act (ADA) was passed in 1990 and prohibits discrimination on the basis of disability in all facets of public life. Specifically, the five titles of the ADA promote inclusion in employment, state and local government, public accommodations, telecommunications, commercial facilities, and transportation. The ADA does not actually address the issue of voting. However, its amended version, the ADA Amendments Act (ADAAA) of 2008 is interpreted by many as promoting voting rights for the disabled. This is because it clarifies the meaning of Title II to include voting as a "service program or activity provided by a public entity" (ADAAA s. 794(b)). The ADAAA's implied sanction of voting for those with developmental disabilities can be seen as a catalyst for finding reasonable accommodations for their enfranchisement.

Our nation has a complicated history when it comes to voting rights. The reality is that in 1789, "[w]e the people," as mandated by the Constitution was roughly 6% of the population, comprised of white males, who either owned property or paid property taxes. Even though the United States was organized as a representative democracy in its formative years, a little under 95% of the population did not have the right to vote. Fortunately, after much struggle, Amendments to the Constitution and federal legislation ever so gradually expanded the franchise. The aftermath of the Civil War brought the 13th Amendment, which outlawed slavery in 1865. The 14th Amendment granted due process and equal protection to all natural born and naturalized citizens, and the 15th Amendment granted the right to vote to African American males. World War I and the women's suffrage movement led to the 19th Amendment which granted women the right to vote. The civil rights movement led to the 24th Amendment which abolished poll taxes in 1964. The Civil Rights Act of 1964, and the Voting Rights Act of 1965 (VRA) abolished literacy tests and residency requirements. Finally, amidst protests from the Vietnam War, the 26th Amendment lowered the voting age to 18 in 1971. Today, in 2022, there still exist struggles and hard-fought legislative battles, at the federal, state, and local levels to ensure equity and representation for all citizens in our democratic process.

8.2 Autistic Adults and the Right to Vote

If, as is correctly suggested above, the ADAAA of 2008 confers the right to vote to individuals with disabilities, an examination of current law and policy will determine if this extension of the franchise to autistic adults has been successful, and if not, what changes must occur.

Prior to examining current law and policy, one must consider what characteristics of an autistic individual serve to create a state of disenfranchisement. In other words, most citizens aged 18 and older, in the United States, not currently or formerly incarcerated or lacking mental capacity have the right to vote. So, why are some autistic individuals denied the right to vote? The answer lies in a determination of mental incapacity, whether or not an individual is unable to make their own decisions due to illness or disability. Historically, it was believed that these potential voters could be susceptible to voter fraud, in that their caretakers or family members would vote for them.

In fact, the concept of an "educated electorate" as a prerequisite necessary for a successful democracy was a widespread belief and pervasive in the writings of the founding fathers (Monticello 2021a). Thomas Jefferson was particularly passionate about education and he devoted much of his life after his presidency to developing a system of public education in Virginia. He poignantly commented, "Whenever the people are well informed, they can be trusted with their own government" (Monticello 2021b). Jefferson proposed a system of broadening education by taxing the rich to educate the poor to enable the common man "to vote understandingly." However, his educational vision was far from universal and only included white males. Paradoxically, efforts to broaden voter inclusion in American democracy have necessarily come at the cost of lowering the median educational level of the voting population (Levine 2003). Literacy tests, one of the many so-called "Jim Crow Laws," were used as a litmus test for voting, under the guise of ensuring an informed electorate. In reality, such restrictions were aimed at curtailing African–American voting and may have had the consequence of limiting voting for developmentally disabled citizens.

Fortunately, the elimination of literacy tests in the landmark Voting Rights Act (VRA) 1965, other civil rights precedents, and the ADA and ADAAA have laid the groundwork for courts to re-examine voting rights for the mentally and developmentally challenged. Constitutional scholars have argued that universal suffrage is guaranteed by the "equal protection" provisions of the 14th Amendment. The concept of "one man one vote", albeit originally coined in a decision on congressional redistricting, is another catch phrase which embodies this principle (Macker 1984). This tension of individual rights versus the common good is at the core of what makes our democracy work and involves a requisite balancing of the harm of the individual right against the common good of society. In the case of an autistic adult, the question turns on whether allowing an autistic individual to exercise the right to vote will bring more harm than good. In other words, will that action work to the detriment of the public good? According to one commentator, "It seems unlikely that extending the franchise more broadly to persons with mental disabilities would alter the outcome of many elections." (Appelbaum 2000).

Several court cases have weighed in on this question. In general, the federal courts have determined that any adult citizen who has the ability to cast a ballot and have that ballot counted has the right to do so. In Doe v. Rowe, the state of Maine was sued for prohibiting persons under guardianship for mental illness from registering to vote (Doe v. Rowe 2001). The federal district court agreed that Maine had a "compelling state interest in ensuring that those who cast a ballot have the mental capacity to make a decision by being able to understand the nature and effect of voting itself" (Doe v. Rowe 2001). However, the court maintained that Maine could exclude an individual incapacitated only to the extent that he or she lacked understanding of the "nature and effect of voting" as determined by a "clear and fair standard" (Doe v. Rowe 2001). In the absence of such a standard, denial by the state was considered a violation of the equal protection statute of the 14th Amendment, as well as Title II of the ADA (Disability Justice 2021).

Two court decisions in 2012 involving the Minnesota State Constitution were decided similarly. In *Minnesota Voters Alliance v. Ritchie*, the court noted that the Minnesota Constitution states that individuals under guardianship cannot vote (Minnesota Voters Alliance v. Ritchie 2012). However, a subsequent statute by the legislature noted that persons under guardianship are presumed to retain the right to vote unless otherwise denied by a court. A few months later in *re Guardianship of Brian W. Erickson*, the precedent of *Doe v. Rowe* was applied, and the court ruled that the Minnesota Constitution's denial of voting rights violates equal protection and due process. This meant that all those under current guardianship at that time retained their right to vote. Moreover, the ruling stated that all future guardianship proceedings include an *independent evaluation of the voting ability of each ward* (Disability Justice 2021).

These court decisions have stressed the need for a low threshold and tend to favor efforts to enhance and protect widespread voter participation with minimal restrictions. Moreover, they have served as an impetus to update many antiquated state constitutional and statutory provisions regarding mental incapacity and voting. The state of Illinois has addressed this question and is one of eleven states with no restrictions on voting for those with cognitive or mental disabilities. However, nine states—Alabama, Louisiana, Massachusetts, Minnesota, Missouri, South Carolina, South Dakota, Utah and Virginia—still have constitutional limitations on voting for anyone declared to be cognitively or mentally impaired (Mathis 2020). Many states are in the process of reviewing and updating their laws to reflect the more permissive standards encouraged by the courts.

Although the courts continue to encourage preservation of the secret ballot for disabled voters, they have recognized that this idea is often not feasible. The (VRA) 1965 and the Help America Vote Act of 2002(HAVA) legislated accommodations for blind, disabled, and illiterate voters. They are permitted to have an assistant of their choice accompany them in the voting booth. The only restriction is that the assistant cannot be the voter's employer or a union representative (Commonwealth of Pennsylvania 2021). Still, in the case of the autistic voter, concerns are often raised regarding the possibility that a parent or guardian acting as an assistant could unduly influence or even coerce their ward's vote. This would in effect result in the guardian voting as a proxy, which is voter fraud and would mean that the guardian is effectively voting twice.

Elections are administered on the state and local level in the United States, and as such there is no uniform method of voting. Roughly half of states use optical scan ballots, which are paper ballots that a voter marks and then places in a scanner that will indicate an over vote (a voter has voted for more than one candidate in a race) or an under vote (a voter has not voted for candidate). More than a quarter of states use electronic or touch screen voting (Direct Recording Electronic Systems (DREs)) with a simultaneous printed record called a Voter Verified Paper Audit Trail (NCSL 2021) . Provisions of HAVA have banned older technologies, such as lever or punch card systems as a requisite of receiving funding in federal elections and require that all precincts have at least one machine accessible to disabled voters. The American ballot is often long and complicated since officials are elected at the federal, state, and local levels of government.

The legal age of transition from childhood to adulthood is also called the "age of majority" (Hamilton 2016). This term is descriptive because it defines the age when an individual becomes legally responsible for the majority of his or her decisions. Parents or guardians are presumed to be their decision makers until children reach this crucial turning point. In the United States, the age of majority was 21 from colonial times until 1971 (Hamilton 2016). At that time, public sentiment arose for lowering the voting age to 18 to match the age of conscription and the age 19 Vietnam War draft lottery. The 26th amendment was ratified on July 1, 1971, and lowered the voting age for federal elections to 18. Over the past 50 years, almost all states have lowered their ages of voting and majority to 18 or 19. Some have also linked majority to graduation from high school.

While most 18-year-olds are celebrating their high school graduations and emancipation to majority, autistic 18-year-olds often become the subject of petitions for guardianship, due to having reached the age of majority and out of concern for an individual that might lack the capacity to undertake personal, medical, or financial decisions on their own behalf. For a detailed description of guardianship, please see Doyle, Chap. 1.

With the logarithmic growth of the neurosciences over the past 50 years, autism is now recognized to be a spectrum disorder with numerous neurological etiologies. That is, the hypothesized cause of autism is an underlying organic brain dysfunction which can be traced to a myriad of neuroanatomical, neurophysiological and neurochemical anomalies resulting in impaired brain maturation. Furthermore, the etiologies of autism spectrum can often be identified and studied with neuroimaging, electroencephalography, and genetic assays. Numerous pharmacological, behavioral, and educational interventions have been developed which can improve outcomes. Management is a team effort involving the cooperative efforts of parents, educators, therapists and physicians. Successful interventions can be measured by "normalization" of behaviors resulting in improved learning, cognition and developmental progress (Dawson 2008).

8.3 Guardianship and Autism

Despite our best efforts, the prevalence of autism spectrum disorders continues to increase and in the United States is estimated at 1 in 59 (Baio et al. 2014). Many of these children will reach the age of 18 with persistent cognitive and behavioral impairments which will affect their transition to majority. Some argue that lack of normal brain maturation in effect creates an implicit condition of chronic and refractory childhood which could preclude voting eligibility. Disenfranchisement in such instances should not be construed as judgmental or punitive but rather as based on scientific data and historical precedents, as well as religious and ethical concepts. Guardianship measures are designed to protect the health and wellbeing of the adult autistic citizen. However, if conceived as a public health measure, guardianship also protects the general public from the consequences of an autistic adult's inability to make rational life decisions.

The role of medical and mental health experts in guardianship proceedings cannot be underestimated. In Cook County, Illinois, a qualified physician must complete a detailed medical form verifying the respondent's incapacity. This medical form specifically inquires whether the respondent is **totally** or **partially** incapable of making **personal** and **financial** decisions. Some may argue that an individual who is **totally** incapable of making such meaningful decisions, could also be incapable of making the **political** decisions required for voting. There are also those that argue that the level of capacity for political decision making should be held to a much lower standard than meaningful personal or financial decisions (Okwerekwu et al. 2018). However, the Cook County guardianship physician report form does not address this crucial question, nor do most guardianship forms.

The physician who verifies that an 18-year old autistic citizen is sufficiently disabled to require guardianship bears a heavy responsibility since the process will, in effect, result in a permanent restriction of the individual's civil rights. Society should expect that such physicians have the proper specialty training and credentials to diagnose and manage autism spectrum disorders. Typically, the appropriate specialists include pediatric neurologists, child psychiatrists and psychologists, and developmental pediatricians. Furthermore, it should be recognized that autism is a relatively new category of developmental disability with a definition that is still evolving and a prognosis that is highly variable. On the other hand, simply justifying the disenfranchisement of autistic adults under guardianship on the basis of their prolonged state of minority may be an inadequate argument. Some political scholars have argued that children ***should*** be given the right to vote (Demeny 1986). They reason that earlier engagement in the political process would increase the rights of children and enhance their legitimacy as political constituents.

8.4 Alternative Solutions to Ensuring the Right to Vote for Autistic Adults

Having a lack of decisional capacity or being declared *non compos mentis* (not of sound mind), in matters related to health, safety, monetary control, and housing, has resulted in many autistic adults being placed under guardianship. Although individuals might be placed into guardianship due to lack of capacity to make certain decisions, the effect of guardianship can extend to all aspects of a ward's life. In other words, though an autistic adult might lack the mental capacity to make sound financial decisions, the full effect of a guardianship will often extend well past financial matters. The right to vote is one such area that is negatively impacted and is quite often an unintended consequence (Vasilogambros 2018). As of October 2020, 13 states have laws barring individuals under guardianship from voting; four states bar individuals deemed *non compos mentis* from voting; seven states use such outdated language as "idiots" and "insane persons" to bar individuals from voting; and 22 states and the District of Columbia only bar an individual from voting if a court has determined that the individual lacks the specific capacity to vote (Mathis et al. 2020).

From the beginning of this nation's history the right to vote has been considered a cherished right of citizenship. In fact, since 1787, when the U.S. Constitution was first signed into law, there has been a struggle, which continues today, to expand and provide equal access to the franchise to as many eligible voters as possible. The United States is after all a representative democracy, which means that our government is intended to represent and give a voice to all of our citizenry, not a select privileged few. As discussed above, the rights of disabled individuals to vote have been considered on the federal level since the VRA 1965, the National Voter Registration Act of 1993, the ADAAA 2008, and the HAVA. 2002. But, how do these seminal pieces of voting rights legislation address mental disabilities and the right to vote? The key seems to be in the distinction that mental illness and mental disability are different than mental incapacity to vote and that different standards apply. For instance, the VRA allows individuals with disabilities to appoint someone to assist in voting as well as requiring that states not treat individuals with mental disabilities differently than the general voting age population; the National Voter Registration Act permits assistance and services to all people with disabilities; the ADA provides that individuals with disabilities have an equal opportunity to vote; and finally the HAVA provides for accessibility for individuals with disabilities (Okwerekwu et al. 2018).

All of these provisions under federal law have been undertaken in an effort to ensure equal access and opportunity to the electoral process for all. How then do we address and ensure the rights of autistic adults to exercise their franchise? The answer lies in the severity of autism in the individual as well as the areas in which an autistic adult might lack decisional capacity. One might query what is the difference in understanding political issues between the average voter and an autistic adult? Political understanding is not a requirement to vote, so why should it be for those with mental disabilities? In fact, international studies have shown that voting is a key aspect of citizenry for psychiatric patients and that the act of voting creates a sense of order and belonging (Okwerekwu et al. 2018). Ultimately, the success of our democracy is measured by the participation of all members of our citizenry. Civic engagement is key to our civil society as is evidenced by the centuries-long, ongoing battle to provide equitable access to our electoral process. The following discussion offers alternatives and solutions to individuals who have lost the right to vote as a consequence of being placed under guardianship or some other legal process. Our purpose is not to endorse one method over another, but rather to stoke thoughtful discussion and engagement for proponents and advocates of voting for autistic adults.

8.5 "Proxy" Voting for Severely Autistic Adults

Currently proxy voting is illegal in all public elections in the United States. Simply put, it is considered voter fraud for a voter to vote twice. However, the concept does have historical precedent. It was utilized in the American colonies to facilitate voters in frontier areas who could not easily travel to distant polling places. Proxy voting was also allowed for some of the northern troops in the Civil War. Canada allows proxy voting in its remote territories as well as for military personnel and prisoners of war. In the United Kingdom a voter may appoint a proxy if he or she has a valid reason for missing an election (Gov.UK 2021).

Political decision making, particularly in today's highly polarized society, can be overly stressful to anyone and may be an unreasonable expectation for a severely autistic adult. Indeed, some argue that severe autism can preclude the capacity and cognitive ability to understand the process of voting, and thus such individuals should not be allowed to vote. Others may argue that the process can be modulated through the mechanism of guardianship. Accordingly, proxy voting by guardians with input from the severely autistic ward could be examined as a viable means of enfranchising severely autistic adults. In reality, as there is no effective way to regulate assisted voting once the guardian and ward enter the voting booth and in the case of mail in ballots, it is possible that a form of proxy voting is already occurring. The danger in these actions is that proxy voting is currently illegal and some might consider the guardian, depending on the circumstances, to be voting for themselves and their ward. As such, it would therefore be more reasonable to acknowledge this situation, that guardians, with the input of their wards, are providing assistance to vote and legitimize it. The current status quo is comprised of antiquated, dysfunctional and often unenforceable regulations which vary from state to state. It intimidates rather than encourages the autistic voter, often leading to the least desirable outcome—abstaining and staying home.

The guardian is legally and ethically bound to act in the ward's best interests and is already serving as the ward's proxy in virtually all aspects of adult decision making. By this way of thinking it is only logical that the guardian should assume the role of political proxy as well. As such the guardian would have the moral imperative to vote in the best interests of the autistic ward. The guardian's right to the ward's proxy, with input from the ward, could be legally codified in the guardianship document. This would serve as a reminder to be vigilant on behalf of the ward's political and social rights and to vote for those individuals and policies which would protect those rights. In this manner, it might be possible for the unfettered voice of the severely autistic citizen to be legitimately expressed and included in the American democratic process.

8.6 Limited Guardianship

If an autistic adult who desires to participate in the electoral process lives in a state where guardianship or conservatorship status is creating a statutory barrier to voting, there are solutions in place to rectify the loss of franchise. First, if the guardianship is not yet in place, one should consider preserving the right to vote for a ward. A type of limited guardianship should be considered. While most applications for guardianship do not address the right to vote, the American Bar Association, through its Commission on Law and Aging, adopted policy, in 2008, and which the Uniform Law Commission incorporated, in 2017, as part of its Uniform Guardianship, Conservatorship, and Other Protective Arrangements Act, Section 310, that state guardianship laws should explicitly state that the right to vote is retained in guardianship proceedings, and must therefore be specifically removed, by a court of competent jurisdiction, as part of the proceeding (Sabatino 2020). This approach to guardianship seems logical and better suited to address the true needs and limitations of a prospective ward, and, as Sabatino states, "[i]n a time when the franchise is increasingly under siege, small advances represented by this kind of legislation make a huge difference" (Sabatino 2020). If a guardianship already exists, steps can be taken to amend the document to restore the ability to vote to the ward.

8.7 Supported Decision Making

One alternative to guardianship proceedings, whether limited or not, is that of Supported Decision-Making (SDM). SDM allows individuals with disabilities to retain their decision- making authority with the "support" of trusted loved ones and advisors, hence the name. The underlying concept is not unlike how most people live their lives. Whether we make decisions about our work, financial matters, or even our personal lives, who amongst us has not sought the counsel or advice of family, friends, or professionals as we determine our next step? SDM just formalizes the process to empower individuals with disabilities to make decisions without stripping them of those rights through a guardianship or conservatorship. To be clear, SDM will not work for all individuals with disabilities; it is merely a less restrictive option that will work for some. In addition to creating an environment of support, in the context of voting rights, SDM will not adversely affect an autistic individual's ability to vote.

8.8 Conclusion

The dialogue surrounding the right to vote for autistic citizens is important and long overdue. The rights of citizens in the United States are enshrined in the Constitution and its preamble, "[w]e the People," which in a representative democracy means all of the people, including autistic citizens. Going forward, we must consider and respect all of the sacrifices and hard fought victories achieved through the VRA and the ADA, which seek to provide equal access to the polling place to individuals with disabilities. Our laws should be drafted in a manner that seeks inclusion of as many eligible voters, as opposed to exclusion. As we have seen in the past, the path to voting rights can be complicated and is often two steps forward, and sometimes one or two steps back at the same time. But, we persevere because we know that civic engagement is the cornerstone of our democracy. We know that we should consider the rights of all citizens to vote and that we cannot leave our marginalized and disadvantaged citizens behind. In fact, we should work harder to ensure that their interests and voices are not silenced and acknowledge that "[t]his citizenship-oriented approach to care not only respects a patient's health, but also their rightful place in society" (Okwerekwu et al. 2018). Toward the important end of ensuring that autistic adults, along with all other individuals with disabilities, are given their rightful opportunity to cast a ballot, we must confront the obstacles that exist, however uncomfortable they may be to discuss, and work together to find solutions that will not only empower autistic adults, but will also ultimately inure to the benefit of our civil society.

References

ADA Amendments Act 2008 (US).

Americans with Disabilities Act 1990 (US).

Appelbaum, P. S. 2000. 'I Vote. I Count': Mental disability and the right to vote. Psychiatric Services 51(7): 849–863. https://doi.org/10.1176/appi.ps.51.7.849.j.

Ashley Noble. 2016 Dependent health coverage and age for healthcare benefits. *National Conference of State Legislature*. https://www.ncsl.org/research/health/dependent-health-coverage-state-implementation.aspx. Accessed 5 Apr 2021.

Baio, J., L. Wiggins, D.L. Christensen, et al. 2014. Prevalence of autism spectrum disorder among children aged 8 years. *Autism and Developmental Disabilities Monitoring Network* 67 (6): 1–23.

Commonwealth of Pennsylvania, Voting in PA. https://www.votespa.com/Voting-in-PA/Pages/default.aspx. Accessed 5 Apr 2021.

Dawson, G. 2008. Early behavioral intervention, brain plasticity, and the prevention of autism spectrum disorder. *Development and Psychopathology* 20: 775–808. https://doi.org/10.1017/S0954579408000370.

Demeny, P. 1986. Pronatalist polices in low-fertility countries: Patterns, performance, and prospects. *Population and Development Review* 12: 335–358.

Disability Justice, The Right to Vote. https://disabilityjustice.org/right-to-vote/. Accessed 4 Apr 2021.

Doe v. Rowe. 2001. 156 F.Supp.2d 35.

Evans, B. 2013. How autism became autism. *History of the Human Sciences* 26 (3): 3–31. https://doi.org/10.1177/0952695113484320.

Gov.UK. 2021. How to vote. https://www.gov.uk/how-to-vote#voting-by-proxy. Accessed 5 Apr 2020.

Hamilton, V.E. 2016. Adulthood in law and culture. *Tulane L. Rev.* 91: 55.

Help America Vote Act of 2002 (US).

Levine, R. H. 2003. The (Un)Informed electorate: Insights into the supreme court's electoral speech cases. Case Western Reserve L. Rev. 54(2): 225.

Macker, A. 1984. One Man, One Vote—Yes or No? *New York Times*. https://www.nytimes.com/1964/11/08/archives/one-man-one-voteyes-or-no.html. Accessed 4 Apr 2021.

Mathis, J., et al. 2020. Vote. It's your right: A guide to the voting rights of people with mental disabilities, 13–14. https://disabilityjustice.org/right-to-vote/. Accessed 5 Apr 2021.

Minnesota Voters Alliance v. Ritchie. 2012. 890 F.Supp.2d 1106.

Monticello. 2021a. Research & Education, https://www.monticello.org/research-education/. Accessed 3 Apr 2021.

Monticello. 2021b. Extract from Thomas Jefferson to Richard Price. https://tjrs.monticello.org/letter/118. Accessed 4 Apr 2021.

National Conference of State Legislators, Elections and Campaigns. https://www.ncsl.org/research/elections-and-campaigns.aspx. Accessed 5 Apr 2021.

Okwerekwu, J.A., et al. 2018. Voting by people with mental illness. *Journal of the American Academy of Psychiatry and the Law* 46 (4): 2. https://doi.org/10.29158/JAAPL.003780-18.

Sabatino, C.P. 2020. Guardianship and the right to vote. *Human Rights* 45 (3): 17.

Shiner, K., and L. Ochs. 2000. Making exceptions to universal suffrage: Disability and the right to vote. In *Encyclopedia of criminology and deviant behavior*, ed. C. E. Faupeland, and P. M. Roman, 179–183

U.S. Const. amend. XIV.

U.S.C. § 794(b).

Vasilogambros, M. 2018. Thousands Lose Right to Vote Under 'Incompetence' Laws, Pew Charitable Trusts. https://www.ncsl.org/research/health/dependent-health-coverage-state-implementation.aspx. Accessed 5 Apr 2021.

Voting Rights Act of 1965 (US).

Chapter 9
Autism, the Criminal Justice System, and Transition to Adulthood

Kenneth A. Richman, Katrine Krause-Jensen, and Raffaele Rodogno

Abstract The criminal justice system is set up for the purpose of regulating people's behavior. If an individual violates a criminal norm, sanctions should reflect that person's mental capacity in understanding what they did was legally wrong. When an autistic individual commits a crime, questions may be raised as to the responsibility of key social/state actors for failing to provide structures that would facilitate accepted behavior in this special category of citizens. Many of the infractions that autistic individuals are likely to commit come as a result of failed interactions with the wider neurotypical society as well as with law-enforcement officials. If the general public were more sensitive and educated about some of the issues raised here, and if (parts of) the public realm were less stressful and more autism friendly, there may well be fewer problematic incidents involving autistic people.

9.1 Introduction

With fully grown bodies, access to adult activities, and still-developing executive function skills and social understanding, it is not surprising that young adults are the group most likely to be arrested (Office of Juvenile Justice and Delinquency Prevention 2019). As young people transition to adulthood, they lose the support offered by schools and, eventually, parents. When young adults are autistic, the challenges increase. Police officers and autistic citizens can fail to understand each other, and can have difficulty predicting what the other will do. Officers can misinterpret autistic speech as uncooperative or disrespectful; autistic people can misunderstand or have difficulty complying with expectations of officers, or fail to appreciate an officer's authority to enforce compliance. The same applies in court settings. Research suggests that not only autistic people and their parents, but also police and legal

K. A. Richman (✉)
Center for Health Humanities, MCPHS University, 179 Longwood Avenue, Boston, MA, USA
e-mail: kenneth.richman@mcphs.edu

K. Krause-Jensen · R. Rodogno
School of Culture and Society, Aarhus University, Aarhus, Denmark

N. Elster and K. Parsi (eds.), *Transitioning to Adulthood with Autism: Ethical, Legal and Social Issues*, The International Library of Bioethics 91,
https://doi.org/10.1007/978-3-030-91487-5_9

professionals are often dissatisfied with their interactions (Crane et al. 2016; Maras et al. 2017). Here we examine this topic from the perspective of philosophical ethics and law, with emphasis on moral responsibility and justice.

An important aspect of this discussion has to do with whether a person is responsible for what she did. When we say that a person should not be held fully responsible for an action, this does not mean that the action should be allowed or that the action is not a problem. We only mean that the individual should not be blamed or punished. It might still be imperative for someone—the individual herself or others—to take steps to avoid it happening again.

Our discussion makes no claims about how likely it is that autistic individuals will commit crimes. It is generally accepted that autism makes people more likely to be victims than perpetrators of crime, and there is no conclusive evidence that autism increases the likelihood of criminal behavior (Heeramun et al. 2017). We certainly do not want any reader to fear or try to control people just because they are autistic. But, like members of other groups, some autistic people will sometimes commit criminal acts. How, if at all, should their autism affect the response? To get started, we offer three real-world examples.

9.2 Examples

Manny

Our first example is from a mother who gave us permission to share her son's story. Her son, whom we will call Manny, is an intelligent 16-year-old autistic male. Manny has been bullied at school, and fears being bullied again. He has no real friends, although he has a great wish to have some, and spends time with peers who engage in risky and socially questionable behavior.

Manny's mother asks him about news that students are illegally selling the tobacco product snus at Manny's school. Manny denies knowing anything, and excuses himself abruptly. A few days later, a police officer comes to their home. Manny admits delivering snus and collecting money for the dealers. He knew it was illegal, but wanted to be involved with peers and was happy to pass on the money he collected without keeping any. The police offered not to put the incident on Manny's record if he named everyone involved, which he did.

After some time, one of the dealers texted Manny. This dealer had a car trunk full of snus and marijuana, and believed the police were suspicious. Manny could have the illegal goods for free so the dealer wouldn't get caught with them. Manny considered accepting the offer so he could make friends by giving the goods away. He thought this would be OK because he would not be selling anything. Luckily, he explained this thinking to his mother, who discouraged him.

Manny's mother believed her son felt compelled to do anything to fill his deep need for peer relationships, much as someone might steal if there were no other way to get food. Manny did not understand that he was being exploited. He had difficulty seeing what was relevantly similar about selling the substances and distributing them for free. He also did not appreciate the potential long-term consequences of having a criminal record.[1]

Reginald "Neli" Latson

Neli Latson is a young, autistic Black man with an IQ of 69 (Marcus 2014). In 2010, Neli was outside waiting for the public library to open when a neighbor called the police to report a suspicious person. When an officer tried to question and frisk him, Neli became agitated and aggressive, and the officer was injured (O'Dell 2016). Neli was informed he was "under arrest for refusing to provide his identity," and eventually convicted of "malicious wounding on a law enforcement officer and assault on a law enforcement officer" (Epps 2015). While in jail, Neli was put in solitary confinement, where his mental health and functioning deteriorated.

Neli served two years in prison, and was later transferred to a community-based residential facility. He was re-arrested after another altercation with an officer who was attempting to restrict his movement. At one point he was shot with a stun gun and then strapped to a chair for hours (O'Dell 2016). He spent another year in isolation. In January 2015, Neli was granted a conditional pardon which required him to remain in prison for another six months (Fain 2015).

It seems likely that racial bias played a role in what happened to Neli. Knowingly or not, race may have shaped why someone was bothered by his presence outside the library to begin with, and why the officer felt the need to engage with him physically. Other cases involving autistic Black young men have also ended badly (Sitz and Mesner-Hage 2020).

Nick Dubin

Nick Dubin is an autistic author and advocate who has written at length about his experience with the law (Nick's case is described in greater detail in the chapter authored by his father Larry Dubin). Not long after he earned a doctorate in psychology, Dr Dubin (Nick) was assessed using the Vineland Adaptive Behavior Scale, a tool widely used to evaluate people with developmental differences. Nick's scores indicated a psychosocial age appropriate to a "preadolescent" (Attwood et al. 2014). Based on the gap between his verbal and nonverbal functioning, Nick was identified as having nonverbal learning disability (NVLD) (Attwood et al. 2014).

Curious and concerned about his sexuality, Nick collected a variety of pornographic images from the internet. Some of these involved young children. Nick writes that he understands now that these images and their production were harmful and illegal. When he first viewed them, however, he did not see himself as different from these children. He saw himself as their peer, and was unable to discern from the images that the children were being exploited or harmed. Nick's apartment was raided by the FBI. Nick's parents, therapists, and lawyers supported him through the traumatic process of interrogations, forensic neuropsychology assessments, and court appearances. The court accepted the findings that Nick poses no danger and

---

[1] Manny's story has some similarities with what happened to Jesse Snodgrass (cf. Erdely 2014).

that he did not understand the implications of his actions. Unfortunately, Nick is now a lifetime felon and permanently on the sex offender registry (Attwood et al. 2014).

9.3 Values and Dilemmas

Topics requiring ethical discussion generally involve dilemmas—values that conflict or must be balanced against each other. What values are relevant here? What do we care about when it comes to criminal justice and autistic young adults? In law enforcement and criminal justice, relevant values include fairness, attention to facts, and respect. Respect is owed to innocent civilians, offending civilians, victims, officials, and communities. Respect for individuals, their freedom, and their privacy can conflict with protecting those same individuals and others from harm. Fairness and respect themselves require balancing component values.

The decision of whether to hold someone responsible sits on a key dilemma between respect for an individual's agency and compassion for that individual's limitations. While holding someone responsible for an offense generally comes with blame and the potential for punishment,[2] treating someone as not responsible can exclude that person from participation in significant human interactions and undermine their own sense of themselves as agents.[3] The following discussion should be considered in light of these values.

The remainder of this chapter addresses four aspects of the encounter with the criminal justice system:

1. Autistic individuals' understanding of and ability to comply with legal expectations
2. Interactions between autistic individuals and law enforcement
3. Assessing whether an autistic individual should be found guilty of an offense
4. Appropriate response or punishment for those who are guilty.

9.4 Understanding and Complying

We will draw from a variety of sources to highlight a few ways that autism can make it harder for autistic individuals to know what is expected and behave accordingly. A general range of differences are understood to be characteristic of autism (Fletcher-Watson and Happé 2019). It is worth emphasizing that these characteristics apply to individuals in different measures and combinations, so that autism is not so much a spectrum as a distinctive constellation of skills and experiences in each person (Hearst 2015).

---

[2] Some approaches allow responsibility without moral blame (cf. Pickard 2004).

[3] David Shoemaker discusses the cost of exclusion in an unpublished manuscript (Shoemaker 2019).

Autistic individuals tend to have difficulty understanding the experiences of other people, including predicting their behavior and expectations.[4] This could be due to a primary issue with theory of mind. It could also be due to lower general orientation toward social facts, resulting in a small inductive base for learning social patterns (Fletcher-Watson and Happé 2019). Autistic individuals may miss contextual cues (Vermeulen 2013) or not shift attention to salient facts due to monotropism, which is the tendency to allocate attention to an atypically narrow range of interests (Murray et al. 2005). We see some of these tendencies in our examples. The result can be interpersonal conflict, failure to understand when romantic attention is unwanted, or behavior associated with stalking (Stokes et al. 2007). It is easy to understand how these challenges could cause young people like Manny to choose illegal ways to meet deeply felt social needs.

Intense sensitivity to visual or auditory stimuli (Markram and Markram 2010) can make some autistic people extremely uncomfortable. For instance, some autistic individuals have told us that, for them, being touched by another person is unbearable, even like being burned by acid. This could make someone unable to remain quiet, to speak, to stay in place, or to move away even when required to do so. Consider that a neurotypical individual might be similarly unable to control responses to an explosion, terror attack, or fire.

Stimming behaviors, such as flapping or rocking, can be crucial for maintaining emotional regulation and feelings of safety. Autistic author Fergus Murray connects stimming to monotropism:

> It is easier for autistic people to process one channel at a time. … Often, if we get overloaded, it helps to have controlled or predictable input. Stimming, flapping, rocking and humming provide something we can do and feel without having to think about it, and can make it much easier to filter, to focus on something else, or to deal with feelings (Murray 2019).

To those unfamiliar with this phenomenon, stimming can at times also make it seem that an autistic individual is willfully refusing to comply with the demands of law enforcement or other authorities, and can appear threatening.

Some autistic authors use the word 'inertia' to explain the autistic experience of being stuck—difficulty initiating action, even action that the person needs or wants to do. Karen Leneh Buckle identifies several contributory factors, including planning (executive function), focus (cognitive flexibility/monotropism) , initiative, and motivation (Buckle 2019). Inertia can occur even with respect to matters deeply connected to a person's values. On a broad, second-order level the person cares about caring; in the moment, the first-order, on-the-ground caring is not happening. But autistic individuals can also get stuck and fail to act on matters that they do care about in the moment. Some of these matters can involve responsibilities to others, where failure to act (or to speak) can have legal consequences.

---

[4] This is sometimes attributed to a mismatch between autists and typical social environments rather than any deficit in the autist. Self-styled "Guerilla Aspie" Paul Wady likes to say "We have empathy for our own kind."

We see that some autistic characteristics can make understanding and complying with social and legal expectations harder.[5] The next section discusses challenges arising from interactions between autistic individuals and law enforcement officials.

9.5 Navigating Encounters

Being different makes people vulnerable to discrimination, distrust, or even physical harm. For autistic individuals, this is further complicated because autism can be an "invisible" difference. If someone is blind, this is generally apparent to sighted people around them. Some autistic people are different in ways that are as obvious as being blind. Others show their autism in ways that are clear, but only to those with relevant insight or experience. Still others may be autistic in ways that are not usually noticeable by others but become apparent in situations that reduce available cognitive resources (e.g., when the person is stressed, excited, tired, or engaged in a complex task). This variability can cause uncomfortable surprises for others.

These issues point to what Damian Milton terms "the double empathy problem:" neurotypical people can have difficulty understanding autistic individuals just as autistic individuals can have difficulty understanding neurotypical people (Milton 2012). Double empathy is central to how autism can complicate the workings of criminal justice. Anyone faced with behavior that they cannot predict or that fails to fall into expected patterns is likely to feel threatened, and if law enforcement is involved it is likely that someone is already feeling threatened.

Disclosure can help. Parents can explain to passersby that a child who is stimming or whose clothes are inside out (perhaps to avoid scratchy tags) is autistic (Cobb 2018). Autistic people can carry disclosure cards, and some have advocated for an autism designation on drivers' licenses to facilitate interactions with police (Torres 2019). But while there is increasing understanding of autism, we might still wonder: When we disclose to a community member that a person is autistic, what can we expect that person to know as a result? What can we expect them to do differently?[6] At this point, our expectations should be limited. News stories and television shows are contributing to awareness, but autism sensitivity is in early stages. Practical knowledge about autism is not yet part of the broad social or health literacy expected in communities. Furthermore, autistic people may not think to disclose, or may, for various reasons, choose not to disclose.

Another relevant issue for law-enforcement officers is the co-occurrence of autism and intellectual disability (ID). While "earlier epidemiological reports indicated that as many as 70% of autistic individuals had co-occurring ID," more recent reports, though contested, suggest that "ID was present in as few as 30% of" autistic children. (Thurm et al. 2019). The disparate estimates are partly explained by similarities in how autism and ID are manifested. In Thurm et al.'s deficit-based description,

[5] Members of other groups will have different challenges.

[6] Question suggested by Joel Anderson.

"because many of the social communication deficits that define ASD [autism] represent a failure to acquire developmentally expected skills, these same deficits would be expected to occur to some extent in all individuals with intellectual disability (ID)" (Thurm et al. 2019). Even assuming that the lower estimates were correct, however, there still is a large gap between them and the estimated 1% incidence of ID in the wider population (McKenzie et al. 2016). Ideally, law enforcement officers should be aware that rates of ID are higher in the autistic population and should be prepared to assess and respond to this.

Our case examples describe some situations in which autistic young people might encounter law enforcement officers. The wallet card offered by AANE (the Asperger/Autism Network) to help when autistic individuals need to interact with police lists some of the autistic tendencies that can derail these encounters. This card states that the holder might:

- "Panic if yelled at, and lash out if touched or physically restrained.
- Misinterpret things you tell me or ask me to do.
- Not be able to answer your questions.
- Appear not to be listening or paying attention.
- Tend to interpret statements literally.
- Appear rude or say things that sound tactless, especially when anxious or confused.
- Have difficulty making eye contact.
- Speak too loud, too soft, or with unusual intonation." (AANE Asperger/Autism Network 2019).

These tendencies, if unexplained, could cause a situation to escalate, as it did for Neli Latson (discussed above). Because these behaviors could be interpreted as resistance, the wallet card states clearly "I would like to cooperate."

The card also provides ways for first responders to facilitate cooperation.[7] It could be hard for a first responder to stop to read such a card in an emergency. However, first responders who are familiar with autism can make some adjustments quickly to keep the encounter safe and effective for everyone. Resources and training for this are increasingly available (National Autistic Society 2017).

Once the initial encounter has been navigated, autism can impede efforts to determine relevant facts. Witness interviews and interrogation of autistic suspects require alternative approaches. First, the setting of the interview can be a significant factor. Sensitivity to lighting, sounds, and even smells can make it impossible for some autistic individuals to participate effectively. These can be profoundly uncomfortable or just impossible to ignore, so that they occupy cognitive resources needed to respond in expected ways. Many problematic sensory stimuli can easily be eliminated or reduced once identified. When autistic individuals find the environment tortuous or too distracting, addressing these issues is not unfair special treatment, but a requirement for respect, due process, and fact-seeking.

[7] These include explaining who you are, calling a contact listed on the card, avoiding touching or restraint, and giving very clear instructions (AANE Asperger/Autism Network 2019).

Even where the environment is conducive to exchange of information, an autistic person may misunderstand the nature of the exchange or what is at stake. For instance, even after being escorted out of a high school classroom in handcuffs, autistic student Jesse Snodgrass asked "Am I getting in any trouble?" (Erdely 2014). More than neurotypicals, autistic individuals can require explicit explanations of what is happening and what is expected of them.

Certain types of questions that are usually appropriate in these situations can lead autistic people to appear to confess to acts they did not commit, or to appear uncooperative (Crane et al. 2015). In the UK, the National Autistic Society's (NAS's) "Autism: a Guide for Police Officers and Staff" gives this example: "asking, 'Has your laptop got anything on it about plans for any terrorism acts?' is likely to elicit agreement, as a web browser or a text editor could be used to plan anything" (National Autistic Society 2017). This guide also advises against leading questions, and statements with tag questions ("You went to the shop, didn't you?"), which could also lead to false agreement. It notes that other common question types could lead to false 'no's.' For instance, if an interviewee is explaining what happened at an earlier time, the interrogator might say "so now we are in your apartment?" This could be confusing because the interrogator wants to confirm the sequence of past events but uses the present tense to say something that is, in the present, clearly false.[8]

The "spikey profiles" of some autistic individuals, such that the same person can have very strong cognitive skills in some areas and very weak skills in others, can lead to confusion about what to expect from them. When people are knowledgeable and articulate about many things, it's easy to assume that they also have easy access to social insights and unfairly blame them when their actions or answers fail to take these into account.

In the UK, the Police and Criminal Evidence Act requires the presence of an "appropriate adult" for questioning "a juvenile or vulnerable person" (Home Office UK 2019). The law's definition of vulnerability includes autism-relevant characteristics such as "difficulty understanding or communicating effectively about the full implications for them of any procedures and processes connected with" their interactions with the police (Home Office UK 2019). Involving an appropriate adult can be an excellent way of facilitating effective interactions.

9.6 Assessing Guilt

Once the initial encounters are done and an autistic individual has been charged with a crime, what role could autism play in determining whether the defendant should be found guilty? The following discussion relies on some concepts from English common law as codified in the American Model Penal Code, or MPC (American Law Institute 2008). These legal concepts parallel ethical ones in many ways, but here we focus on legal issues. We are not defending the legal categories as correct or

[8] See Maras (2020) for a useful and relevant discussion of related matters.

ideal, only using them as guideposts for thinking about how autism intersects with some legal criteria relevant to culpability.

Substantial capacity

First, let's consider the following clause from the MPC:

> A person is not responsible for criminal conduct if at the time of such conduct as a result of mental disease or defect he lacks substantial capacity either to appreciate the criminality [wrongfulness] of his conduct or to conform his conduct to the requirements of law (American Law Institute 2008).

Autism is not a "mental disease or defect," but might it affect substantial capacity to appreciate wrongfulness or conform conduct? One of us has argued elsewhere that autism can reduce a person's access to information relevant to the wrongness of an action (Richman 2017; Richman and Bidshahri 2018). Such information can include the experiences of others, and what alternative actions were available.

The Reporter's comment on MPC 4.01 (1) remarks that: "An individual's failure to appreciate the criminality of his conduct may consist in a lack of awareness of what he is doing or a misapprehension of material circumstances, or a failure to apprehend the significance of his actions in some deeper sense." Autism doesn't cause someone to be unaware of what they are doing. However, autism may account for some misapprehension of social information, as in the case of Nick Dubin, or failure to apprehend the significance of actions, as with Manny. These failures (or difficulties) are not the kind of global incapacity that comes with severe psychosis or an epileptic seizure. They are limited in scope, and, as we see with Nick Dubin, seem to have more to do with "reasons blockage" (Richman 2017) than with the ability to appreciate the wrongness of actions once the morally relevant features are apparent. That is, there may be some information that would cause a neurotypical person to change her behavior, but that might not be accessible to an autistic individual. We do not blame people for failing to respond to facts that are not available to them.

Atypical cognitive styles can contribute to this phenomenon. Typically developing children and adults have a tendency to "process incoming information for meaning and gestalt (global) form, often at the expense of attention to or memory for details and surface structure" (Happé and Frith 2006). This particular cognitive style may help explain skills in generalizing, i.e., in recognizing situations that are different in some respects as nonetheless belonging to the same (proto)type. This capacity might well be at play when we place distinct particular actions under the same category, as, for example, when we infer from the fact that a certain action is wrong that another, relevantly similar action is also wrong. The cognitive style that characterizes autism is different in this respect, as it tends to focus on detail as opposed to the general or global. This may in turn result in a difficulty in inferring the wrongness of one action from the wrongness of another similar action in spite of a general capacity to discern right from wrong.

Of our few examples, only Neli Latson appears broadly unable to conform his conduct to the requirements of law. This is likely not a function of autism alone. His intellectual disability appears to have intensified his difficulty understanding and communicating about his situation, his inability to predict what will happen in the novel situation of the first encounter with police, and what must have been severe discomfort in response to unwanted touching and restraint. Neli's intellectual disability is global in a way that Nick's NVLD is not. This makes it more obvious how Neli could lack substantial capacity with respect to the interactions leading to his arrest.

Section 4.3 of the MPC requires that an intention to rely on a defense of mental disease or defect be filed at or around the time of a not guilty plea. This suggests that if a person lacked substantial capacity, that person is not a candidate for another defense. A finding that someone lacked substantial capacity might thus be understood as an exemption, not an excuse. It is a finding that the person was, at least at that time in respect to that action, outside the community of those who are even candidates for responsibility. Despite this treatment in the MPC, since autism per se appears to cause specific challenges rather than global incapacity, we suggest that when autism is exculpatory, it is more likely to justify an excuse for a particular action than an exemption that puts the autistic person outside the community of responsible agents.

Actus reus

Under common law traditions, criminal culpability generally requires both *actus reus* (guilty act) and *mens rea* (guilty mind). Failure of one or the other would be a legitimate excuse for many types of offenses.[9] The *actus reus* must be voluntary rather than, for example, a spasm or reflex. Could autism be relevant to whether an action is voluntary?

As discussed above, someone who can generally conform behavior to the requirements of law might have a sudden and involuntary response to touch or other stimuli, and that response may look to others like voluntary violence. Challenges with inhibition, an executive function that can be reduced in autism, may be relevant. Stimming behaviors may also be difficult to stop if they are part of how an autistic person maintains equilibrium or relative calm. Issues with sensory overload and high levels of anxiety may also arguably decrease the level of voluntariness of one's (re)actions. These phenomena can raise questions about whether the *actus reus* requirement for culpability was satisfied.

Mens rea

Someone can satisfy the *mens rea* requirement for criminal culpability by acting "purposely, knowingly, recklessly, or negligently, as the law may require, with respect to each material element of the offense" (American Law Institute 2008). *Purposely* and *knowingly* require intentions (purposely) or expectations (knowingly) that the harmful results of a voluntary action will occur. 'Recklessly' applies when a person "consciously disregards a substantial and unjustifiable risk" (American Law Institute 2008). Autism hardly seems exculpatory when someone has these mental states with respect to harm that the person knows is wrong.

[9] Culpability for strict liability crimes does not require *mens rea*.

Autism might, however, make it harder to determine what a defendant knew, expected, or consciously disregarded. It is characteristic of autistic individuals (especially young autistic persons) to have difficulty with perspective-taking. This applies to their own earlier selves (Happé 2003). By around age four, typically developing children understand that others might have false beliefs that contradict the child's own true beliefs (Baron-Cohen et al. 1985). Autistic individuals tend to catch up on this ability in well-defined tasks that can be taught, but can continue to show difficulties in real-life situations (Klin et al. 2002). Those who do poorly at these tasks with others may also forget that they themselves had false beliefs at a previous time (Happé 2003). This can be very problematic when it comes to assessing culpability. Consider an autistic person who attacks someone in her apartment thinking that the person is a dangerous intruder, and who then learns that the "intruder" was her roommate. We can speculate that, if the autistic person struggles with theory of mind issues, she may falsely report that she believed it was her roommate all along.[10] This could lead to a false guilty verdict.

Negligence "involves a gross deviation from the standard of care that a reasonable person would observe in the actor's situation" (American Law Institute 2008, 2.02(2)(d)). The reasonable person standard is intended to offer an objective way of assessing what a person ought to have known about or done in response to some risk. Variation has been allowed for children on the basis that:

> Children are less able than adults to maintain an attitude of attentiveness toward the risks their conduct may occasion and the risks to which they may be exposed. Similarly, children are less able than adults to understand risks, to appreciate alternative courses of conduct with respect to risks, and to make appropriate choices from among those alternatives (American Law Institute 2010, p. 116).

Autistic adults, even young adults, are not children. They can, however, have similar challenges with attentiveness to, understanding, and responding to risk. It is appropriate, then, that legal scholars continue to argue for personalized application of the reasonable person standard: "The reasonable person standard, traditionally derived from an aggregate relevant pool, would be replaced by the 'reasonable you' standard—a personalized command that is based on information about *this* actor's specific characteristics" (Ben-Shahar and Porat 2016, p. 629). Given the great variety in the autism constellation, a "reasonable you" standard may offer the best promise of fairness in determining whether a person has been culpably negligent.

---

10 This suggestion is based on extrapolation from data involving children (Happé 2003) showing challenges with attributing false beliefs to the earlier self and data showing that, with substantial variation, some autistic adults perform poorly at theory of mind tasks (Brewer et al. 2017). Future data might show that the type of error described is quite unlikely.

9.7 Shared Responsibility, Structuring Causes

Behavior is shaped by social structures much as mobility is shaped by the physical environment. This is easiest to see with young children (who depend on adults to structure activities and social interactions to facilitate a successful day) or drivers (who depend on road design and signs to travel safely). When an autistic individual commits a crime, questions may be raised as to the part of responsibility that might be attributed to key social/state actors for failing to provide structures that would facilitate accepted behavior in this special category of citizens. Many of the infractions that autistic individuals are likely to commit come as a result of failed interactions with the wider neurotypical society as well as with law-enforcement officials. If the general public were more sensitive and educated about some of the issues raised here, if (parts of) the public realm were less stressful and more autism friendly, there may well be fewer problematic incidents involving autistic people.

The social conception of disability can provide illumination here. According to that concept, disability is a state of society (not of individuals) that puts some people at a disadvantage (Silvers 1996). If disadvantage arises from a state of society, the community as a whole bears responsibility for the consequences. When the disadvantage consists in extra difficulty conforming to legal expectations, there may be instances when it is reasonable to assign blame for transgressive behavior quite widely.

In a recent dialogue with the autism community in Aarhus, Denmark, an autistic autism consultant suggested that local municipalities offer "autistic ambassadors" as a social service. These specially trained helpers would have the task of accompanying groups of autistic individuals on, say, a night out, functioning as an interface between the autistic individuals and their environment, ensuring smooth transitions on public transportation, in public houses, cinemas, shops, etc. Similarly, one may argue that government bodies should ensure that the general public and its officers have a basic understanding of autism. This would arguably be as necessary to guarantee the equality and dignity of autistic individuals as the provision of wheelchair access to public spaces is necessary to guarantee the equality and dignity of those who cannot walk. If provision of such services could be shown to be a legitimate claim and be linked to diminished violations by autistic individuals, societies that could provide these services but failed to do so may indeed be understood as sharing in the responsibility for such violations.

9.8 Determining an Appropriate Response or Punishment for Those Who Are Guilty

Legal punishment is commonly understood as "imposing *deprivation* ("hard treatment") on someone, in a manner that conveys *censure*" (Von Hirsch and Ashworth 2012, p. 17). The idea of censure is quite central here. Unlike other methods for the regulation of behavior such as for example the imposition of a tax, penal sanction involves reprobation and blame. At its heart, then, we find a form of moral communication between the state as the representative of society and the act's perpetrator or wrongdoer. By visiting hard treatment upon the offender, the state sends the message to the offender (as well as to society at large) that, for example, harming someone is wrong and will not be tolerated. In this communication, the offender is treated as a moral agent, that is, "someone who is offered moral reasons for specified choices, for he is assumed capable of comprehending and acting on such reasons" (Von Hirsch and Ashworth 2012, p. 17). This, of course, is not to say that consequentialist aims such as harm prevention are not also at play in punishment. Yet sanctions that do not involve censure as described here will fail to treat offenders as persons or moral agents, and would rather treat them as beings that need to be "restrained, intimidated, or conditioned into compliance" (Von Hirsch and Ashworth 2012, p. 18).

This conceptualization of legal punishment nicely explains why expressions of guilt and remorse on behalf of the offender during trial or in the process of parole granting may mitigate or shorten the punishment, as these emotions are taken to signal that the offender has recognized and repudiated the wrongness of their conduct that the punishment is meant to convey. Yet the very same feature so elegantly explained by this view of punishment is likely to discriminate against individuals like those on the autism spectrum who have difficulties with social communication and with understanding and expressing emotions. In fact, one may wonder how autistic individuals receive and understand the whole idea of punishment as moral communication of censure. In the other direction, judges and juries may fail to appreciate an autistic person's expression of remorse, resulting in an unfairly harsh sentence.

These worries notwithstanding, this view inspires a plausible theory of sentencing that revolves around the principle of proportionate, deserved sentences: penalties are graded according to the degree of reprehensibleness, that is, the harmfulness and culpability, of the actor's conduct, with a view to communicating censure rather than to matching the level of deprivation imposed on the offender to the level of suffering of the victim ("pay back" or lex talionis). Proportionate sentencing is not confined to the realm of philosophical ideas but has inspired sentencing policies in the United States, Finland, Sweden, Canada, New Zealand, and England (Von Hirsch and Ashworth 2012, p. 1). This view is interesting here for it prescribes sentencing policies that are particularly attentive to the case of juveniles and, as we shall argue, to autistic juveniles. In short, the idea is that the same criminal act should receive a lesser sentence when committed by a juvenile as opposed to a mature person and that for two reasons: (i) diminished culpability due to the juvenile's diminished cognitive and volitional capacities; and (ii) increased punitive "bite." The rationale behind (i) is already clear from our discussion above. Let us, then, focus on (ii).

As a general rule, a given penalty is considered to have greater punitive bite when suffered by a child or a juvenile than when suffered by an adult. That's because the former are less psychologically resilient and their punishments interfere more with opportunities for education and personal development (Ball et al. 1995, p. 116;

Zedner 1998, p. 173). Now consider the evidence cited by Johnston in her discussion of "just deserts" for offenders with "severe mental illness" (Johnston 2013, p. 151). Autism is not a mental illness, but autistic individuals tend to share relevant vulnerabilities. Compared to typical people, those with the kinds of "cognitive and behavioral limitations" (Johnston 2013, p. 151) that tend to be experienced in autism and mental illness (i) are more vulnerable to bullying and predation inside (as well as outside) prison and (ii) have a harder time coping with prison structures and rules, hence incurring relatively more disciplinary violations (as in the case of Neli). In short, they are more susceptible to serious harm in prison. This extra susceptibility should be factored into the sentences of autistic juveniles (and adults) if we do not wish them to suffer undeservedly more onerous punishments than their peers who are not affected by these differences or limitations (Johnston 2013). Autism should then be considered as a mitigating factor in determining appropriate sentences.

9.9 Conclusion

Autism can be relevant to all facets of an autistic person's engagement with the criminal justice system. Being autistic can make it harder to appreciate and conform to social and legal expectations, and can pose challenges for the interactions with law enforcement that follow social disturbances or accusations of illegal behavior. Autism can also provide good reasons for finding that someone should not be punished for offending behavior, and good reasons for deviating from sentencing standards used for neurotypical offenders. While these considerations are not specific to young people transitioning to adulthood, they are most relevant to that age group because young adults are the most likely to offend and be arrested.

We hope these findings are helpful for families, schools, the law enforcement community, and others. They point to a wide range of topics for future work. For instance, to develop usable models of the "reasonable you" standard, we might want to learn more about how specific types of neuropsychological profiles affect ability to perceive and respond to morally/legally relevant information. Community views on sentencing may be relevant. We may also want to see how the considerations treated here fit into ongoing philosophical discussions of moral responsibility. The concept of "answerability" discussed by David Shoemaker and others (Shoemaker 2015) may be promising in this context. Answerability, as opposed to simple blameworthiness, may provide a framework for retaining as much as possible the idea that autistic individuals are moral agents—members of the moral community—while recognizing vulnerabilities and mitigating factors. As always, a primary challenge is to provide an analysis that makes sense for a wide enough range of autistic profiles while also allowing for individualized application, all with respect and while honoring the autistic experience. We hope this chapter has moved the dialogue a bit further in that direction.

References

AANE Asperger/Autism Network. 2019. Wallet Card. https://www.aane.org/resources/wallet-card/. Accessed 30 March 2021.

American Law Institute. 2010. *Restatement of the law, third: Torts: Liability for physical and emotional harm: Restatement*, vol. 1. Philadelphia, PA: American Law Institute Publishers.

American Law Institute. 2008. *Model penal code*. Buffalo, NY: William S. Hein & Co.

Attwood, T., I. Hénault, and N. Dubin. 2014. *The autism spectrum, sexuality and the law: What every parent and professional needs to know*. London: Jessica Kingsley Publishers.

Ball, C., K. McCormac, and N. Stone. 1995. *Young offenders: Law, policy and practice*. London: Sweet & Maxwell.

Baron-Cohen, S., A.M. Leslie, and U. Frith. 1985. Does the autistic child have a "Theory of Mind"? *Cognition* 21 (1): 37–46. https://doi.org/10.1016/0010-0277(85)90022-8.

Ben-Shahar, O., and A. Porat. 2016. Personalizing negligence law. *New York University Law Review* 91 (3): 627–688.

Brewer, N., R.L. Young, and E. Barnett. 2017. Measuring theory of mind in adults with autism spectrum disorder. *Journal of Autism and Developmental Disorders* 47 (7): 1927–1941. https://doi.org/10.1007/s10803-017-3080-x.

Buckle, K.L. 2019. Autistic inertia: Why do we get stuck? Paper presented at the Autism Show, Manchester, UK.

Cobb, M. 2018. We had a great day at the park with our autistic son, until someone called the police. https://www.washingtonpost.com/news/parenting/wp/2018/02/08/we-had-a-great-day-at-the-park-with-our-autistic-son-until-someone-called-the-police/?utm_term=.9930c9cc07fa. Accessed 30 March 2021.

Crane, L., et al. 2016. Experiences of autism spectrum disorder and policing in England and Wales: Surveying police and the autism community. *Journal of Autism and Developmental Disorders* 46 (6): 2028–2041. https://doi.org/10.1007/s10803-016-2729-1.

Crane, L., L. Henry, K. Maras, R. Wilcock. 2015. Police interviewing of witnesses and defendants with autism: What is best practice? http://network.autism.org.uk/knowledge/insight-opinion/police-interviewing-witnesses-and-defendants-autism-what-best-practice. Accessed 30 March 2021.

Epps, K. 2015. Reginald "Neli" Latson case: Wounding charges advance in Stafford. *The Free Lance Star*. https://fredericksburg.com/local/reginald-neli-latson-case-wounding-charges-advance-in-stafford/article_cf08ce79-9eba-5e24-82a4-84a1c15f261d.html. Accessed 30 March 2021.

Erdely, S.R. 2014. The entrapment of Jesse Snodgrass. Rolling Stone. https://www.rollingstone.com/culture/culture-news/the-entrapment-of-jesse-snodgrass-116008/. Accessed 30 March 2021.

Fain, T. 2015. *McAuliffe, from hospital, pardons autistic man*. Daily Press. https://www.dailypress.com/government/local/dp-mcauliffe-from-hospital-pardons-autistic-man-20150120-post.html. Accessed 30 March 2021.

Fletcher-Watson, S., and F. Happé. 2019. *Autism: A new introduction to psychological theory and current debate*. New York: Routledge.

Happé, F. 2003. Theory of mind and the self. *Annals of the New York Academy of Sciences* 1001 (1): 134–144. https://doi.org/10.1196/annals.1279.008.

Happé, F., and U. Frith. 2006. The weak coherence account: Detail-focused cognitive style in autism spectrum disorders. *Journal of Autism and Developmental Disorders* 36 (1): 5–25. https://doi.org/10.1007/s10803-005-0039-0.

Hearst, C. 2015. Does language affect our attitudes to autism? https://www.autismmatters.org.uk/blog/does-language-affect-our-attitudes-to-autism. Accessed 30 March 2021.

Heeramun, R., et al. 2017. Autism and convictions for violent crimes: Population-based cohort study in Sweden. *Journal of the American Academy of Child & Adolescent Psychiatry* 56 (6): 491-497.e492. https://doi.org/10.1016/j.jaac.2017.03.011.

Home Office (UK). 2019. *Police and criminal evidence Act 1984 (PACE): Code C revised*. London: The Stationery Office.

Johnston, E.L. 2013. Vulnerability and just desert: A theory of sentencing and mental illness. *Journal of Criminal Law and Criminology* 103 (1): 147–229.

Klin, A., et al. 2002. Visual fixation patterns during viewing of naturalistic social situations as predictors of social competence in individuals with autism. *Archives of General Psychiatry* 59 (9): 809–816. https://doi.org/10.1001/archpsyc.59.9.809.

Maras, K.L., et al. 2017. Brief report: Autism in the courtroom: Experiences of legal professionals and the autism community. *Journal of Autism and Developmental Disorders* 47 (8): 2610–2620. https://doi.org/10.1007/s10803-017-3162-9.

Maras, K. 2020. Cognition in autism: Implications for practice in the criminal justice system (and beyond). Paper presented at the Autistica Research Festival. https://www.youtube.com/watch?v=bvfHmCrPBLw&list=PLg_hTtp1fDqqn0qLCwbbxIWTnYcyQ1uJA&index=2. Accessed 30 March 2021.

Marcus, R. 2014. In Virginia, a cruel and unusual punishment for autism. Washington Post. https://www.washingtonpost.com/opinions/ruth-marcus-in-virginia-a-cruel-and-unusual-punishment-for-autism/2014/11/14/9d7f6108-6c3b-11e4-b053-65cea7903f2e_story.html. Accessed 30 March 2021.

Markram, K., and H. Markram. 2010. The intense world theory—a unifying theory of the neurobiology of autism. *Front Hum Neurosci* 4: 224. https://doi.org/10.3389/fnhum.2010.00224.

McKenzie, K., et al. 2016. Systematic review of the prevalence and incidence of intellectual disabilities: Current trends and issues. *Current Developmental Disorders Reports* 3 (2): 104–115. https://doi.org/10.1007/s40474-016-0085-7.

Milton, D.E.M. 2012. On the ontological status of autism: The 'Double Empathy Problem.' *Disability & Society* 27 (6): 883–887. https://doi.org/10.1080/09687599.2012.710008.

Murray, F. 2019. Me and monotropism. *The Psychologist* 32: 44–49.

Murray, D., M. Lesser, and W. Lawson. 2005. Attention, monotropism and the diagnostic criteria for autism. *Autism* 9 (2): 139–156. https://doi.org/10.1177/1362361305051398.

National Autistic Society. 2017. Autism: A guide for police officers and staff. https://www.autism.org.uk/products/core-nas-publications/autism-a-guide-for-criminal-justice-professionals.aspx. Accessed 30 March 2021.

O'Dell, L. 2016. Lawsuit says Virginia jailers abused autistic inmate. Fredericksburg.com. https://www.fredericksburg.com/news/state_region/lawsuit-says-virginia-jailers-abused-autistic-inmate/article_bec2d0a4-0814-11e6-9aed-9fdd95f3b78c.html. Accessed 30 March 2021.

Office of Juvenile Justice and Delinquency Prevention. 2019. OJJDP Statistical Briefing Book. https://www.ojjdp.gov/ojstatbb/crime/ucr.asp?table_in=1. Accessed 30 March 2021.

Pickard, H. 2004. Responsibility without blame: Therapy, philosophy, and law. *Prison Service Journal* 213: 10–16.

Richman, K.A. 2017. Autism and moral responsibility: Executive function, reasons responsiveness, and reasons blockage. *Neuroethics* 11 (1): 23–33. https://doi.org/10.1007/s12152-017-9341-8.

Richman, K.A., and R. Bidshahri. 2018. Autism, theory of mind, and the reactive attitudes. *Bioethics* 32 (1): 43–49. https://doi.org/10.1111/bioe.12370.

Shoemaker, D. 2015. *Responsibility from the margins*. New York: Oxford University Press.

Shoemaker, D. 2019. Disordered, disabled, disregarded, dismissed: The moral costs of exemptions (Unpublished Manuscript).

Silvers, A. 1996. (In)equality, (Ab)normality, and the Americans with disabilities act. *Journal of Medicine and Philosophy* 21 (2): 209–224.

Sitz, L.H., Mesner-Hage, J. 2020. How a black autistic man is serving 10 years in prison for a car crash. Washington Post. https://www.washingtonpost.com/video/local/how-a-black-autistic-man-is-serving-10-years-in-prison-for-a-car-crash/2020/09/10/7f86aed2-5a58-475d-a806-3957ee3bdb2c_video.html. Accessed 30 March 2021.

Stokes, M., N. Newton, and A. Kaur. 2007. Stalking, and social and romantic functioning among adolescents and adults with autism spectrum disorder. *Journal of Autism and Developmental Disorders* 37 (10): 1969–1986. https://doi.org/10.1007/s10803-006-0344-2.

Thurm, A., et al. 2019. State of the field: Differentiating intellectual disability from autism spectrum disorder. *Frontiers in Psychiatry* 10 (526): 1. https://doi.org/10.3389/fpsyt.2019.00526.

Torres, J. 2019. Family pushes for autism symbol to be added to New York Driver's licenses. ABC News. https://abc7.com/5694497/. Accessed 30 March 2021.

Vermeulen, P. 2013. *Autism as context blindness*. KS: AAPC Publishing.

Von Hirsch, A., and A. Ashworth. 2012. *Proportionate sentencing: Exploring the principles*. New York: Oxford University Press.

Zedner, L. 1998. Sentencing young offenders. In *Fundamentals of sentencing theory: Essays in honour of Andrew von Hirsch*, ed. Ashworth, A., M. Wasik, A. Von Hirsch. Oxford: Clarendon Press.

Chapter 10
Social Media/Online Behavior and Transition: A Personal Story of an Attorney Father About His Autistic Son and the Criminal Justice System

Lawrence A. Dubin

Abstract This is a personal narrative written by the father of an autistic adult who became enmeshed in the criminal justice system. He writes about their family's experience and offers reflections and recommendations. It is written with the son's permission.

10.1 Introduction

I am a parent of an only child who is an autistic adult. His name is Nick. As Nick was growing up, I never anticipated that I would ever be working on any writing project about Nick's involvement in the criminal justice system. By education and experience, I am a lawyer. After graduating from the University of Michigan in 1966, I practiced law for eight years then became a law professor for the next forty-four years. During those years I also produced public television documentaries, appeared on television as a legal analyst, and wrote legal books about trial practice, the rules of evidence, and the ethical rules for lawyers.

This is our story that began on a day that drastically changed our lives. On October 6, 2010, a beautiful fall morning, I was driving to the university where I work to teach when my cell phone rang. The caller identified himself as an FBI agent. I assumed that he was calling to get a recommendation for a former law student who was applying for a position with his department. I could not have been more wrong.

The agent told me that he and his team were in the process of executing a federal search warrant of my son's apartment. Those words initially made no sense. My son was the most law-abiding person I knew. He was a rule follower, not a rule breaker. He had never been in any trouble with the law. He liked to spend time by himself reading or listening to music. When his peers were out partying or going to school events, he found reasons to avoid those social occasions. Yet he was a personable,

L. A. Dubin (✉)
University of Detroit Mercy, Detroit, MI 48301, United States
e-mail: ladonlow@aol.com

N. Elster and K. Parsi (eds.), *Transitioning to Adulthood with Autism: Ethical, Legal and Social Issues*, The International Library of Bioethics 91,
https://doi.org/10.1007/978-3-030-91487-5_10

likeable, good-looking young man who, at the age of 27, had been diagnosed on the autism spectrum (although at the time the diagnosis was called Asperger's.)

I soon learned that despite Nick's history of law-abiding behavior, he had downloaded illegal images of people under the age of eighteen onto his computer. The day after the FBI search, Nick appeared in federal court for an arraignment on those charges. That day began a twenty-seven-month period of terror that culminated in a plea agreement that would change his status from having successfully overcome a developmental disability to a convicted federal felon and registered sex offender.

10.2 History of Nick's Development

My wife Kitty and I were married in September 1969. She was 23 years old and I was 26. We were both just starting our professional lives. I was working at a law firm and she was teaching at a local college and eventually would become a produced playwright. At that young age, we both felt that we lacked the maturity to take on the demands of parenting. Eight years later, our careers had progressed and Nick, our only child, was born. We were delighted to be parents and anticipated raising him with great joy in our hearts.

Nick was a beautiful baby with a head full of blond hair. We enjoyed putting him in a stroller and walking around the streets of our city, going to parks, and feeding ducks. He started walking before his first birthday. Shortly thereafter, Nick began to behave in an unusual manner. He would jump up and down, flapping his arms as if he had no control over his body.

As a toddler, we took him to parent-child groups where it became noticeable that he had no interest in socializing with other children. There were times he would become very annoyed when approached by other children who wanted to play with him. In groups, he was always on the periphery of the other children who were playing with each other.

At three years old, Nick's language consisted of a few words. He also made up his own version of words that only had meaning to him. We took him to be evaluated by a speech and language clinic at a local hospital and he was diagnosed with aphasia, echolalia along with gross and fine motor delays. He also liked to touch other children's heads, which was not a winning strategy for making friends. Today, the diagnosis would have been that Nick was on the autism spectrum. However, in 1972, the diagnosis of Asperger's (now classified as an autism spectrum disorder) was not one that was recognized until the mid-1990s.

Nick went through his entire public school education with many academic problems. He was classified as a special education student with a somewhat ambiguous learning disability. His speech developed rapidly after speech therapy, which was very reassuring to my wife and me. He had great anxiety in the classroom and difficulty participating in group activities.

Nick was a frustrated student who did not do well academically. Some teachers thought that he did not try hard enough. He was bullied by both fellow students and even some teachers. His art teacher would make fun of his work product in front of the class, informing his classmates that Nick's work was a sample of how their project should not be done. My wife and I made many trips to his school to discuss Nick with teachers, counselors, and even the principal. They simply did not seem to understand that the issues he faced were obstacles to his ability to learn.

Nick seemed to develop certain special interests. He loved listening to music and watching game shows on television, especially *The Price is Right*. Although his gross and fine motor skills seemed to deprive him of playing certain sports (e.g., soccer, baseball), at the age of ten he took a tennis lesson. We soon discovered that a new special interest was born.

For some unexplainable reason, Nick loved playing tennis. He watched every major professional tennis match from the past twenty years, over and over again. His mind became a repository for the collective winning shots of the best professional players in the world. Nick's tennis skills lead him to eventually become an all-state tennis player in high school, the captain of his team and ranked as one of the top players in our four-state division. Yet in spite of his athletic success, he developed no friendships with any of his teammates.

During his adolescence and throughout his high school years, he didn't socialize with his peers. He didn't go to parties or show any interest in exploring his sexuality through relationships. Although he saw many therapists over the years, the fact is that neither Nick nor my wife or I understood why Nick lacked a normal social appetite to be with friends. It simply didn't make sense at the time. Years later the reason became understandable.

10.3 Nick's College Years

Nick always wanted to fit in and be accepted by others. It just had not worked out that way. He decided to go away to college, which seemed like a risky choice, but that's what most of his fellow students were doing and he did not want to be different. He went to a university about 150 miles from our home. He was also selected to play number one singles on the tennis team. After two weeks in his dorm, he demanded to come home and drop out of school. It was too noisy and the socializing was too demanding.

In an effort to avoid an early failure in his academic career, I was able to find him a room in the basement of a private home where he could have peace and quiet. I tried to entice him to finish his academic year by promising him that if he did so, we would go to Los Angeles and get tickets for *The Price is Right*. During the academic year, he drove home every weekend unless he had a tennis match. To his credit, he finished the academic year, played well for the tennis team, and decided the next year to live at home and attend a local university which he graduated from with a BA in Communications. I fulfilled my commitment and Nick and I went to Los Angeles and got tickets to *The Price is Right*. He was selected as a contestant and won $6,000. He spent the funds to buy jazz CD's that were used for his radio program on his college station.

After graduating, Nick decided to obtain a teaching certificate with a major in learning disabilities with the goal of helping children who like him were receiving special education services. He worked on this Master's degree over four years, did exceptionally well in the academic coursework, but after a few weeks of student teaching in a second grade class, decided that he couldn't handle the multi-tasking necessary. Nick agreed with his supervising teacher that being an elementary teacher was not for him. Although he didn't earn a teacher's certificate, he did graduate with a Master's degree in learning disabilities.

With a new direction for his future plans, he applied for admission to a doctorate program in psychology at a local college. He was accepted on the condition that he complete a number of psychology courses. While taking abnormal psychology, he read about Asperger's Syndrome and became convinced that this diagnosis applied to him. To confirm his suspicions he made an appointment with a noted neuropsychologist who did extensive testing and ultimately confirmed that he definitely had Asperger's. The doctor told Nick that with his strong verbal skills, getting a doctorate would permit him to translate what it is like to be autistic to parents, teachers, and even experts like his doctor. Confirming this diagnosis for Nick was very positive. It helped explain all the difficulties he had experienced in his life. He could now understand that his problems were related to neurological issues from birth. Nick vowed that his new goal in life was to help autistic people to better cope with their life challenges. While working on his doctorate, Nick spent 2,000 hours being supervised at a university under a professor who specializes in autism and at a non-profit serving the autism community.

After five years of study, which included writing a successful doctoral dissertation, Nick earned a doctorate in psychology. During these academic years, he became an expert on Asperger's. His expertise lead to publishing contracts for several best-selling books including *Asperger's and Anxiety*, published by Jessica Kingsley Publishers, which has sold over 20,000 copies. These books led to Nick to speak at autism conferences around the country. After all the years of struggle that he endured, he had now achieved his goal of being in a position to help translate what it is like to be autistic to other professionals, teachers, professionals, and to help those who were also autistic.

10.4 Nick, Sexuality & the Criminal Charges

When Nick was arrested at the age of 33, the one thought I had was that I knew he was not a criminal. He was not a predator and was no threat to anyone including children. Yet paradoxically he was charged with very serious federal crimes. During this time, my family was on an isolated island of pain. We did not know anyone else who had experienced the terror of the criminal justice system. During the next few years, as a result of a book Nick co-wrote about his life and experiences in the criminal justice system (with world renowned autism experts Tony Attwood and Isabelle Henault) so many other families contacted us. They all had an autistic son who had been charged with various criminal non-touch sex offenses involving possession of child pornography, stalking, and exposure of private parts.

I reviewed many court files involving autistic men who were charged with a sex-related crime. The forensic reports in these cases as well as many articles written by lawyers, psychologists and social scientists led me to the conclusion that there was a correlation between the developmental disability of autism and the crime charged. The following list is a summary of characteristics attributed to these men that may have led to them unwittingly committing criminal acts without the intent to violate the law or hurt anyone. It is important for criminal defense lawyers to make sure that this information is presented to prosecutors who need to understand this information in the context and purpose of exercising human compassion while seeking a just disposition of a matter.

1. **Autism is a neurological developmental disorder from birth**

An autism spectrum disorder is not a mental illness. This is an important distinction. Psychological developments from birth through adolescence and into adulthood are impacted by the social impediments due to this neurological disorder. The net effect is that Nick and others like him have difficulty experiencing normal social and sexual interactions with other people. The paradox is that in spite of this stunted social/sexual development, their physical bodies with attendant hormones are developing in a normal timetable. Autistic people are sexual people but may not seem that way to others (See Kahn, Chap. 3). The dichotomy of this developmental impediment creates a tremendous gap between their social difficulties and their inner unexpressed sexual thoughts, desires, and feelings.

2. **Many autistic people are average or even above average in intelligence**

Often, there are significant differences among this population in the various types of intelligence. Someone who is a mathematics or computer genius may, at the same time, lack the ability to understand the content of a simple story. The commonality is that a person's general intelligence may be significantly more advanced than their social intelligence, each of which can be measured independently from the other. This means that a person who appears to be highly intelligent in speech and lifestyle might also be at the level of a young child when it comes to understanding social norms and mores. This type of person might confuse a prosecutor who focuses on the intelligence and ignores the significant areas of weakness that more accurately reflect the autism.

3. **The neurology of an autistic person creates deficits in "executive functioning" and "theory of mind"**

A simple description of these terms can be found on the website of AutismSpeaks.org. "Executive Functioning includes skills such as organizing, planning, sustaining attention and inhibiting inappropriate responses." "Theory of Mind is the ability to attribute subjective mental states to oneself and to others" (Begeer 2011). This deficit is sometimes referred to as "mindblindness" which means that an autistic person believes that his thoughts and feelings are also being experienced by other people without being able to recognize the differences that others might have (Rudacille 2011). Hence, an autistic person's ability to engage in normal social and sexual interactions can be significantly impaired by these deficits

These deficits in an autistic person are a result of the wiring of the brain which increases the internal focus on one's thoughts, feelings, ideas and interests derived from his external world. The classic autistic child can be thought of as spinning a top while blocking out his environment. The focus on internal thoughts diminishes one's capacity to understand the emotional needs of others thereby making a successful social connection with other people more difficult.

4. **Autistic people often rely on computers to acquire information on many topics of interest without the need for social interaction**

The computer is the perfect vehicle for a socially inward person to learn information that is normally acquired through interaction with other people. Therefore, sexual knowledge and interest can be easily pursued by viewing images available at no cost on a computer without leaving the privacy of one's own room. To an autistic person, the motive for viewing these images is completely void of criminal purposes.

5. **It is common for autistic individuals to be severely bullied by their peers throughout the childhood and adolescent development**

Many continue to be bullied even as adults by employers who might not be sensitive to their individual needs (See Weitzberg, Chap. 5). The consequence of being bullied throughout their lives causes further social withdrawal and can drive a person into greater social isolation. The computer might become the only way to learn about and experience their sexuality. This dynamic might cause the lack of sexual experience of the autistic person to search out on the computer illegal images not for any illegal thoughts of harming such a person but simply because of the comfort level of the viewer.

6. **Autistic individuals tend to be rule followers and not rule breakers**

Being autistic may cause a person to feel different from others. An autistic person wants to fit in but is confronted by a reality where that is indeed a challenge. So being a rule follower is a compensatory way to not stand out as being different from others.

What I have learned from my son's experience in the criminal justice system is filtered through my lens of having been a lawyer for over fifty years. When I practiced law, I did criminal defense work, representing clients for charges that ranged from drinking and driving to homicide. As a defense lawyer, my job was to protect the constitutional rights of my clients whether I personally believed they were innocent or guilty. That issue was for the jury. As a matter of legal ethics, I was not permitted to put any witness on the stand, including my client, if I had knowledge that perjury would be committed.

As a law professor, I taught legal ethics including the special ethics rules that apply only to prosecutors. In addition to the role of being advocates, there is an additional and very important ethical obligation that prosecutors must meet which is that they must also act like "ministers of justice" and exercise their prosecutorial discretion in a way that will best achieve that goal (Galin 2000). The lawyer who represented Nick had formally been the chief of the criminal division in the office that prosecuted Nick. He had left that office after 35 years of public service. He had never represented a person charged with a crime, in spite of numerous requests to do so, as he had no desire to ever be a criminal defense lawyer. Yet there was one exception that he made. He represented Nick because he strongly believed that Nick should not be prosecuted and instead should be placed into a diversion program.

In the federal system, only the prosecutor, not a judge, has the power to divert a person from the criminal justice system (Bellin 2019). This gives a prosecutor a tremendous amount of discretion in deciding how a case can be resolved. Nick's lawyer believed diversion was necessary for justice to be achieved. Diversion would have placed Nick on an 18-month probationary period terminating without him having any criminal record. This disposition would have recognized that Nick presented no danger to the public while placing him under court supervision to ensure that fact. This process would have protected the public while also permitting Nick to avoid the stigma of being a felon and registered sex offender. Nick's lawyer had great respect for his former office but honestly believed that they "got it wrong" by failing to exercise their discretion as a minister of justice.

Why didn't Nick get diversion? There is no good reason that I can offer. The prosecutors had him evaluated by experts of their own choosing. One expert in particular was employed by the FBI as a neuropsychologist. He read Nick's entire life's medical and psychological history and spent an entire day evaluating him. This neuropsychologist's evaluation recommended to the prosecutors that Nick receive diversion.

The question then becomes trying to understand why prosecutors failed to seek justice through diversion when Nick as an autistic person is charged with a sex crime, has no prior record, and didn't have any intent to harm a potential victim. My answer is that prosecutors often have a conflict of interest that clashes with their duty to seek justice. For example, prosecutors are too often willing to sacrifice justice in order simply to obtain a conviction because more convictions will help them advance in their careers as prosecutors or in running for political office (Bellin 2019). Sometimes the furtherance of other personal interests will conflict with a decision to seek justice. For example, one of my son's prosecutors has made several speeches to FBI agents throughout the country about how people charged with sex crimes are the worst people there are in our country. This prosecutor emphasizes his personal life experience as a child in being sexually abused by a coach over a number of years. His personal interests of seeing all people charged with a sex offense because of his personal history seemed to have conflicted with a more objective view of achieving justice in my son's case in permitting diversion. The prosecutors in

Nick's case acknowledged in their sentencing memorandum to the court that Nick's acts were related to his autism and that he didn't present a danger to the public. Instead of understanding that Nick had a developmental disability through no fault of his own that contributed to his alleged illegal act, the prosecutors disingenuously treated him as if he was an active sexual predator who was dangerous to others in the community. Instead of understanding the nature of the disability and seeking justice, the prosecutors, under the guise of protecting the public, demanded a criminal conviction and registration as a sex offender even though he received probation. In other cases like Nick's, autistic individuals have received lengthy prison terms in addition to having to register as a sex offender. In essence, even though the reason the disabled person committed the criminal act stems from social isolation and fear of social and sexual intimacy, prosecutors prefer to treat them as dangerous predators rather than consider diversion.

Prosecutors often see only a binary choice between an innocent victim and a guilty defendant. When the perceived perpetrator is a person like Nick, the more correct view is that there are two victims and no perpetrators. Nick's victimization is the lack of justice that he received with experts both for the prosecution and the defense who thought diversion was the road to justice. Only the prosecution disagreed from the other experts – even their own.

I want to conclude by offering some brief advice to a variety of stakeholders in cases like Nick's.

To parents

- Recognize your child as a sexual being even though they may show no interest in being sexual (See Kahn, Chap. 3). Their lack of sexual interest may be repressed by their inability to socially relate to others. Seek the necessary services of a qualified therapist with a background in autism spectrum disorders.
- Make sure that your child has an understanding of the dangers of viewing child pornography on a computer and the consequences of doing so. Spare no details. Repeat this message.
- See that your child receives meaningful social skills training to help them develop social awareness.
- Impress upon your autistic child that if ever questioned by police for any reason, they must request that a parent be present. Of course, if necessary, the parent can decide whether a lawyer should be contacted to assert the Fifth Amendment right to remain silent. In other words, the child should not speak to the police without parental or legal guidance.

To therapists with a background in autism spectrum disorders

- In a book written by Nick, entitled, *The Autism Spectrum, Sexuality & the Law*, autism expert and co-author Dr. Tony Attwood (published by Jessica Kingsley Publishers) explained that the deficit of impaired executive functioning can cause an autistic person to have difficulty appreciating the broader perspective of his actions and consequences to himself.

- Dr. Attwood also has indicated that an impaired theory of mind, as commonly associated with autism spectrum disorders, can create difficulty in appreciating the perspective and experiences of another person thereby furthering an emotional detachment while viewing child pornography.
- Therapists need to openly deal with the sexuality of autistic people and explicitly and regularly educate them about the dangers of possessing child pornography, and that doing so can lead to an arrest, a prison sentence, and registration as a sex offender.

To criminal defense lawyers

- Be aware that there are an increasing number of autistic people in the general population which means more of them will enter the criminal justice system. It is incumbent that lawyers understand the nature of autism and how its characteristics might relate to the crime charged. If a client raises concern that he might be autistic, make sure they are evaluated by a competent expert.
- Understand that autistic individuals are often anxious and should be communicated with in a sensitive manner. Consider allowing someone the person trusts to be present during consultations to help with understanding the communications between lawyer and client.
- Prison is the worst place for an autistic person. Whenever possible, strive for a result that can avoid imprisonment.

To prosecutors

- Understand that autistic defendants are generally law abiding and rule following people. The acts that on the surface might be viewed as criminal may have occurred because the developmental disorder lessened their ability to understand that the behavior was wrong or harmful.
- Whenever it appears that an autistic person lacked the intent to commit the criminal act in question and is likely to be educated to not recidivate, consider diversion as the appropriate way to achieve justice.

To judges

- Understand the difference between a developmental disability and a mental illness. Be compassionate when an autistic person is charged with a non-contact sex crime such as possession of illegal images, or a crime reflective of the person's lack of social understanding and norms such as unauthorized touching, disorderly person, or stalking.

To all of the above groups

- Carefully read *Caught in the Web of the Criminal Justice System* written and edited by Lawrence A. Dubin and Emily Horowitz, Ph.D., London, Jessica Kingsley Publishers, 2018. This book presents chapters written by distinguished lawyers and autism experts explaining how certain laws including sex offender registration legislation on a federal and state level were passed based upon moral panic rather than valid underlying data. For example, most people believe that people convicted of a sex offense are likely to recidivate when in fact, sex crimes are one of the lowest rates for recidivism. See the case of Does v. Snyder, 6th federal circuit court of appeals, 2015 for an opinion that discusses the Michigan Sex Offender Registration Act as being punitive and depriving people who have served their debt to society from being able to live a normal life.

References

Begeer, S., C. Gevers, P. Clifford, et al. 2011. Theory of Mind training in children with autism: A randomized controlled trial. *J Autism Dev Disorders* 41 (8): 997–1006. https://doi.org/10.1007/s10803-010-1121-9.

Bellin, J. 2019. The power of prosecutors. *NYU L Rev* 94 (2): 171–212.

Galin, R. 2000. Above the law: The prosecutor's duty to seek justice and the performance of substantial assistance agreements. *Fordham L Rev* 68 (4): 1264.

Gougeon, N. 2010. Sexuality and autism: A critical review of small selected literature using a social-relational model of disability. *Am J Sexu Educ* 5 (4): 328–361.

Parker, M. 2008. Joint study committee on autism spectrum disorder and public safety, 1–3.

Robison, J.E. 2013. Autism and porn: A problem no one talks about. Psychol Today. 6 August 2013.

Rudacille, D. 2011. Mind blindness' affects moral reasoning in autism. https://www.spectrumnews.org/news/mind-blindness-affects-moral-reasoning-in-autism/, Accessed 11 March 2021.

Taylor, K.l., Mesibov, G., Debbaudt, D. 2009. Asperger syndrome in the criminal justice system. www.aane.org/asperger-syndrome-criminal-justice-system, Accessed 11 March 2021.

Chapter 11
A Personal Perspective on Autism and Transition

Allanah Elster

Abstract This is a personal narrative written by a young autistic adult. She describes her childhood without a formal diagnosis of autism and her relationship with her stepbrother who was diagnosed when he was 3. Now that she is recently formally diagnosed with autism, the author reflects on her transition into adulthood, hoping for acceptance and asking that neurotypical people focus on her strengths rather than her perceived deficits or differences.

When I was about 4 years old, I was evaluated by a psychologist in order to join a gifted and talented program at a local top university. My evaluation simply ended with the psychologist telling my mother that they "did not know how to chart my conceptual abilities." So, naturally, I was simply referred to as precocious. My academic propensities weren't all that was "abnormal" about me growing up though. I never quite socially fit in; my interests were hyper-specific and my vocabulary was… unique for my age. Even my style was eccentric. Teachers loved me and called me "an old soul." I was told I would find my place in middle school… then I was told I would find my place in high school… I'm still holding out hope for college. The truth is, though, adults viewed my differences from my peers as positives since these traits made me seem "mature." I, however, only felt isolated. I spent 7 years eating my lunch in teachers' offices because I connected better with the adults than my peers.

Despite my differences, I was never bullied or even that unpopular. According to my peers, I was simply "intimidating." Intimidating is a weird adjective to describe a person because it's like an insult and a compliment all rolled up into one. I was intimidating in that I had clear goals from the start of high school, I quoted philosophers and poets regularly, and I wore suits to school when all my peers were donning pajama pants and Uggs or flip-flops. This made me cool and elusive in some ways, but also unapproachable in others. People feared me in many ways, which I developed

A. Elster (✉)
Columbia University, New York, NY, USA
e-mail: ae2703@columbia.edu

N. Elster and K. Parsi (eds.), *Transitioning to Adulthood with Autism: Ethical, Legal and Social Issues*, The International Library of Bioethics 91,
https://doi.org/10.1007/978-3-030-91487-5_11

into a sarcastic, cold-hearted badge of honor. At the end of the day, however, I felt hurt. I also have always been incredibly direct, for better or for worse. People who got on my nerves would ask "Allanah do you not like me??" While I know logically I should lie, something in me always went with honesty in these situations—"No, I don't like you." "Why do people ask questions they don't want honest answers to?" is a question I continue to ask myself. I used to also be honest about my affection towards people but oddly enough, that was scarier than my direct, yet sometimes harsh honesty. My directness about my affinity towards people scared them off, but my cold, "witty" honesty about things I disliked made people laugh. The thing is, I was never joking. Most people who asked questions like "Do you like me" and received a "No" in response thought it was a joke! Nobody really says no... But I always said what I felt unless of course, I felt something positive that would make me vulnerable. This continues today.

I've grown up deeply immersed in the autism community. I peer mentored students with high assistance needs for 8 years and have grown up with a stepbrother who attends a therapeutic day school for autistic children and adolescents. I always felt a deep connection to my stepbrother. Only two weeks separate our birthdays. He only ever talks about what he wants to talk about–whatever thought jumps into his head. I've always felt like I was actively combatting the urge to do the same. Sometimes at home, I would let my guard down in this regard. If a dinner table topic bored me I would announce "I don't like this topic, it is uninteresting," and I would abruptly get up and leave. I still do. If I were to say that to a group of friends, my concern (and the likely reality) is that I would be ostracized, but my family began to understand my "quirks."

My similarities to my stepbrother were always apparent to me. When someone once asked me if I wished my stepbrother could communicate like "average" people, I asked why shouldn't we all want to communicate like him. His way of living, being honest about his feelings and desires made so much more sense to me as opposed to the confusing landscape of social niceties and mind games that makes up "normal" teenage or even adult communication.

I'm a filmmaker—an artist–which goes against the stereotypical, albeit erroneous narrative of neurodiverse people being science or math geniuses. While I'm not too shabby at calculus, art has always been how I chose to spend my free time and express myself. I often approach social situations in a way that is more scientific than the average person, however. When I first meet somebody, I take in their style, their stance, their tone, and start theorizing about their interiority. Emotions can be difficult for me to understand, so every single external clue I can collect, I compile to inform my interactions. This process is what I believe makes me so good at visual storytelling, but it can also be exhausting. Unlike a novel, making a film only allows you to portray the external factors of a character's thoughts or feelings (unless you employ the dreaded voice-over method... but that's a different conversation). Sometimes, to most comfortably interact with people, I mentally write scripts. I ask myself the same questions I would ask when writing a screenplay. "What is my motivation?" "What is my relationship to the person I'm interacting with?" "What is at stake in this conversation?" Everyday conversations typically don't have objectively high stakes or narratively compelling motivations, but in my mind, answering those questions is a vital part of making sure my thoughts and actions aren't misconstrued.

Some part of me has always known I was neurodiverse, but since I was able to achieve so much and assimilate into mainstream society, my internal struggles were ignored or overlooked for a very long time. During the quarantine of the past year, when my daily battle to figure my peers out was no longer existent, my true self became even clearer to my family. I let down my mask and expressed the thoughts and feelings in my head which previously preoccupied and stifled me. I announced when a sound or a smell made my skin feel itchy and when I wanted a conversation to be over. I dropped the social niceties and finally felt a feeling of relief. However, my family likely felt hurt or concerned that the isolation of COVID was taking its toll. And... I wonder now how, as an adult to take off my mask, and continue to assimilate into the adult world.

I really struggle with empathy and while I can sometimes fake it based on how I think people are supposed to react, I became tired of this act over the last year which was pretty harsh on my family. I have very, very little malice in me at all but I realize that not everyone is as analytical about emotions as I am. Some people just feel hurt or sad even when it is not logical which is really hard for me to grasp. This disconnect was one of the biggest reasons I actually pursued getting evaluated. I realized what I had always feared—my true self, behind all the scripts and pretend niceties, is not someone many people like. That's not to say that neurodiverse people are unlikable or unlovable, but society is not set up to value us for who we are, and so some of us mask. Placing the burden of masking on us is frankly exhausting—something I did not realize until I finally got a break from it, but something I fear I may need to continue as I move on to a college campus, embark on a career, maybe start a relationship, and experience all of the other hallmarks of being an adult. Transitioning from adolescence into adulthood is not easy, especially for those of us who are neurodiverse. As I enter adulthood, I hope that the world around me can accept me and others like me for who I/we are focus on my/our strengths rather than my/our perceived deficits or differences.

Index

N. Elster and K. Parsi (eds.), *Transitioning to Adulthood with Autism: Ethical, Legal and Social Issues*, The International Library of Bioethics 91,
https://doi.org/10.1007/978-3-030-91487-5

CPSIA information can be obtained
at www.ICGtesting.com
Printed in the USA
LVHW082233270422
717440LV00004B/32

9 783030 914868